AYURVEDA

COOKBOOK

A new essential guide to eating and living well with simple tasty recipes, Ayurveda principles, naturally healing your body and increasing your energy with good nutrition

CHAYLA HENCK

INTRODUCTION

Welcome to Ayurveda Cookbook: Ayurveda Recipes to Improve Holistic Health, Wellness and Stress Relieve. The Ayurveda diet was developed thousands of years ago by diligent observation and study by the Indian monks. We were the first to connect the body type to the diet that best supports it.

If you're completely new to Ayurveda, you should realize that it divides people into three main types. Typically, everyone is governed by one type of energy (dosha), another type is the secondary ayurvedic kind.

To figure out which one you are, please review the following descriptions: Vata types tend to be: quick-learning; forgetful; slow circulation, resulting in cold hands and legs; Moody; blasts of tremendous energy in short spurts; impulse; dry hair and skin; scattered; quick-thinking, but often thought-provoking in all directions; loss of daily routine; on the high side; thin-building; quick-moving whey;

Pitta style appears to be: Competitive; Organized; Medium / Strong build; "Hangry" when they miss a meal; Fair-haired and fair-skinned: prone to hot environments; self-confident, assertive, and willing to lead others well; violent and challenging when under tension (to the point of temper tantrums); suffers from skin blemishes (acne, skin cancer, etc.); great public speaking; strong concentration;

Kapha types tend to be: affectionate and acceptable; forgiving; reliable; heavy, but strong; quick to listen and slow to speak; patient; slow and gentle; prone to slow digestion; depressed; possessive (to the point of healing when under stress); extremely calm; firm anchor; soft hair and skin; long-term memory; prone to respiratory ailments; prone to hardened arteries;

If you're still unsure about your form, don't worry about it. Most of the recipes I've chosen will work for any ayurvedic type of recipe. This book will cover recipes from breakfast to dinner, and everything in between. You're sure to find a dish that will cater to your taste buds, whether you're brand new to this lifestyle or if it's been your way of life for many, many years.

Love it!

CHAPTER ONE
OVERVIEW OF AYURVEDA

A philosophy of medicine that originated in India thousands of years ago, Ayurveda is based on the notion that good health relies on the equilibrium of mind, body and spirit.

Considered a complementary approach to health in the United States, Ayurveda focuses on restoring equilibrium in the body through a personalized plan that can include massage, special diets, herbs, aromatherapy and exercise.

Popularity using data from the 2007 National Health Interview Survey conducted by the National Center for Health Statistics (NCHS) Centers for Disease Control and Prevention, 0.1 per cent of respondents have been using Ayurveda over the past 12 months. The percentage of respondents who used Ayurveda was unchanged from the 2002 National Health Interview Survey.1

AYURVEDIC CONCEPTS
According to Ayurvedic theory, everyone is composed of a combination of five elements: air, water, fire, earth, and space. Such elements in the body combine to form three powers, or forces of creation, called doshas: vata, kapha, and pitta.

Though the three doshas have a unique mix, one dosha is typically the most powerful.

In Ayurveda, a person's doshas balance is thought to explain some of their individual differences, and the likelihood of disease. It is assumed that an imbalanced dosha affects the normal flow of vital energy, or prana. The disrupted flow of energy is thought to impair digestion and allow body waste, or ama, to build up which further impairs energy and digestion.

The vata dosha is a combination of air and space. This regulates activity and is responsible for basic functions of the body such as respiration, cell division, and circulation. The body areas of Vata include the large intestine, pelvis, bones, skin, ears, and thighs. People with vata as their key dosha are considered to be quick-thinking, lean, and strong, and prone to nausea, dry skin, and constipation;

The kapha dosha represents the Water and Earth elements. Kapha is thought to be responsible for energy, immunity, and development. Kapha body regions are the fluid in the chest, lungs and spinal cord. Those with kapha are considered to be relaxed as their primary dosha, have a solid body structure and are prone to diabetes, hypertension, sinus congestion and gallbladder issues.

Fire and water are mixed into the pitta dosha. Control of the hormones and the digestive system is thought. Pitta body regions include small intestines, glands of the stomach, saliva, fat, blood, and eyes; It is thought that people with pitta as their main dosha have a fiery temperament, oily skin, and are vulnerable to heart disease, stomach ulcers, asthma, heartburn and arthritis.

A Standard Evaluation An initial evaluation with an Ayurvedic doctor can last an hour or more. In general, the doctor should ask detailed questions about your health, diet and lifestyle. He or she will be listening on your wrists at 12 separate pulse points.

An Ayurvedic doctor also searches at the tongue for hints regarding body locations that may be out of control. We also track the appearance of the head, hair, fingers, and eyes.
After the evaluation the practitioner will determine your unique doshas balance. One dosha is usually dominant and is potentially imbalanced. In fact, the practitioner determines the constitution, or prakut.

RECOVERY STRATEGIES

The doctor usually develops an individualized treatment plan after the assessment, which involves food, exercise, supplements, yoga, meditation, and massage. In general, the treatment plan focuses on restoreing balance to one or two doshas.

- Diet: It may be recommended to take a prescribed diet to balance the doshas of an individual. See a list of foods thought for balancing per dosha.
- Cleaning and detoxification: Fasting, enemas, supplements, and body therapies can be performed.
- Herbal medicine: Turmeric, triphala, ashwaghanda, gotu kola, guggul, and boswellia are examples of Ayurvedic herbs and spices.
- Yoga
- Meditation
- Exercise
- Massage and body treatments: for example, abhyanga, Ayurvedic-style massage, and shirodhara, a therapy involving a stream of warm herbal oil poured on the forehead. Certain therapies for the bodywork include swedana, udvartina, and pindasveda.

- Herbal tea: pitta tea, vata tea, kapha tea Practitioner training There are currently no national certification or licensing standards for Ayurvedic practitioners in the United States or Canada.

Potential safety concerns Ayurvedic products are regulated as dietary supplements in the United States, and are not required to meet the same safety and efficacy standards as drugs.

A 2008 study examined the presence of metals in ayurvedic products sold online, such as lead, mercury and arsenic. Between August and October 2005 the researchers identified 673 products and randomly selected 230 for purchase. Of the 230 items obtained, 193 were received and evaluated for metal presence.

Nearly 21% of the ayurvedic products tested have been found to contain detectable levels of lead, mercury, or arsenic.[2] Research on the efficacy, safety, side effects, and potential drug interactions of ayurvedic herbal products is lacking. Although some research has been done, the architecture of the experiments has generally presented challenges.

The use of such conventional ayurvedic rituals in North America, such as emesis and blood washing, is considered highly problematic and could be dangerous.

BENEFIT IN THE DAILY AYURVEDA ROUTINE

Ayurveda, known to yoga as the "Sister Science," is an ancient, holistic science in nature. Ayurveda's main focus, having been around for more than 5,000 years, is to focus on your life in between the emotional and physical self.

One of the main convictions is that the food we eat has an effect on our overall well-being, and can make us sober or miserable. Essentially, depending on what we bring into our bodies, we can be full of energy and power, or lethargic and run-down. This is known as solution Sattvic.

WHICH ONE IS SATTVIC

Firstly, Sattvic in Sanskrit translates into' pure essence.' Sattvic is a diet based on foods recommended within Ayurveda, and is one of the purest diets that you can take and help you to be your best. This diet is intended to be holistic in nature, meaning it nurtures your mind, body and soul, and is therefore a great support for your practice of yoga and meditation.

Knowing that food is the fuel for our bodies, the peace of mind that it offers us is an additional benefit that correlates with this ancient practice. Ayurvedic practitioners often report being able to concentrate better, sleep better and generally feel less anxious. Here are 10 ways in which Ayurveda will help your everyday life.

1. YOU ARE ENCOURAGED TO LOVE YOURSELF
Ayurveda helps you to find love within yourself rather than being compared to others. It wants you to understand that you are truly unique and designed to be as tailor-made as possible to approach your individual life. This helps you to explore your own needs and to learn, heal and focus on your life.

Ayurveda consists of three main types of body and characteristics of personality which are otherwise known as doshas. The three doshas are Vata, Pitta, and Kapha, and while most people tend to fit a particular dosha, people may often be a mixture of two, with one dosha more prominent than that. See below for a look at your dosha, from Mind Body Green!

VATA: Creative, easy learning and absorbing new knowledge, but also rapid forgetting.
Slender, tall and fast-walker, propensity in cold climates to cold hands and feet and pain, exciting, vibrant, engaging personality
Irregular daily routine, experiencing high energy with a propensity to tire quickly and over-exert in short bursts.

Responding to stress with fear, worry and anxiety, especially when out of balance, is full of joy and enthusiasm when in balance. Tendency to behave on instinct, often have disjointed feelings of driving. Usually have dry hair and dry skin, and don't suck much.

PITTA: Strong and well-built medium physique.
At its best, sharp mind, good concentration, orderly, focused, assertive, self-confident and entrepreneurial. He embracing challenges.
Off balance, aggressive, competitive, demanding and pushy

Great metabolism, great appetite, get annoyed if they've got to miss a meal or wait.

Fair or reddish skin, often with freckles, easily sunburns. Sun, sweaty in sun or hot weather, makes them really sleepy, instantly swell a lot.

Good public speakers, generally good ability to manage and lead but can become authoritarian. Subject to temper tantrums, anger and impatience
Typical physical problems include skin rashes or inflammations, wrinkles, boils, skin cancer, ulcers, heartburn, stomach acid, sleeplessness, swollen or burning hair, etc.

KAPHA: Easy, slow-paced, relaxed. Character affectionate and loving, forgiving, compassionate and non-judgmental, Fidelity, steadiness and efficiency
Physically strong and with heavier, more robust construction
Have the most power of all the constitutions, but it's steady and durable.
Slow speech, reflecting a process of deliberate reflection. Less slow to learn, but exceptional long term memory.

Soft hair and skin, tendency to have large soft eyes and a soft, low voice
It may also suffer from poor metabolism, appearing to be overweight.

Suitable for depression but calm and self-sufficient
Good health and an overall immune system.

Quite peaceful, strive to maintain harmony and peace in the surrounding area. Not easily upset and can be a stabilizing point for others.

Tend to be possessive, to keep things going.

Doesn't really like cool, humid weather

Physical issues include colds and coughing, infections of the sinus, respiratory problems involving asthma, allergy and atherosclerosis (hardening of arteries).

2. OFFERS A NURTURING APPROACH To Be HEALTHY

Ayurveda is all about knowing that your natural state is healthy. If you're in balance with your environment, that's considered optimum health, and the opposite is because you're unbalanced.

For instance, if you feel anxious or suffer from health problems such as constipation or lethargy in general, it's just a matter of being out of balance. Imbalances aren't happening immediately so you have time to prevent or slow down the imbalance cycle. When you know what causes you to feel out of whack, you can simply refer to the suggested foods to be eaten or avoided as per your dosha to start the process of returning to your proper balance.

3. YOU GET A GREATER UNDERSTANDING OF YOUR PLACE IN LIFE

Ayurveda principle is that we are a part of nature. Nature has five elements that include: Space Air Water Fire Earth These elements, their actions, and the presence that they have in your life are a big part of Ayurveda practice.

For starters, Air will show up as high energy and forgetfulness in your body and mind. Fire will manifest as pain, vomiting and vengeance in your body and mind. Earth is linked to your heart, your stubbornness to something and your devotion to others. When you understand which elements present more prominently to you, you will decide which dosha you are and then strive for optimal equilibrium.

4. WE LEARN TO CLEAR UP ENERGY

In this day and age our mental and physical settings are often recalibrated. It is important, as ever-changing beings, to reflect and clarify what does not work for you and your life. It gives space for new things. Cleaning the system with an Ayurvedic-based diet, and regularly cleaning your mind with things like meditation and yoga, will allow you to recalibrate more easily and have greater inner peace access.

5. IT PROVIDES A FULL CIRCLE
Ayurveda PHILOSOPHY reminds you that you are much deeper than your skin. You have an idea, and an aura that can illumine the universe. Ayurveda will keep reminding you that you are more than just muscle and bones, but that you are also a spirit that embodies the elements. While the health benefits will have a positive effect on your physical self, it also puts your mind, body, and spirit together and keeps harmony within all of it. You'll soon begin to see and hear the healing comes from within, beginning with the food that you put in your body.

6. BETTER HEALTH AT A CELLULAR LEVEL
Research shows that Ayurveda can actually be of assistance on a cellular level. It has been suggested that Ayurveda has the potential to actually rebuild cells, demonstrating once again that we have the power to start curing ourselves of certain diseases just by the way we treat our bodies. While research is still under way, the scientific community is hopeful!

7. TOXINS IN THE BODY ARE REDUCED

The founder of the Maharishi Ayurvedic practice states that three different types of toxins are present. The most famous is ama, which is the waste product that builds up from consuming too much of the wrong food in the digestive tract. If not cleaned up, it will build up over time and continue spreading through your system, causing great feelings of unbalance. Different habits within Ayurveda, such as consuming the biggest meal at lunchtime, can keep these contaminants from growing further when the sun is at its peak.

8. STRONGER DIGESTION

The digestive system should improve when you begin eating for your dosha. Certain foods will activate your digestive system during the right time of the day, causing your digestive tract to decrease in toxic build up. This prevents you from feeling lethargic and will cause you to have higher energy levels! Having maximum digestion also helps keep your weight balanced and become less stressed.

9. REDUCED STRESS AND GREATER SENSE OF WELL-BEING

Nutrition affects how you act, to put it simply. If there is no fire in your digestive system, you feel uncomfortable and drained which can turn into negative feelings and ultimately affect how you show up in life. Through adopting a diet specifically tailored to your desires, you will start finding balance in both your body and mind. Again, Ayurveda's holistic approach means it also affects your mindfulness practices positively, helping to reduce overall stress.

10. A STRAIGHT-FORWARD REGIME FOR YOUR DIET

Based on your dosha, the Ayurveda regimen is very straightforward on what you should eat. Guidance on what to eat and when is easy to follow. This no-nonsense method is easy to follow for those who like order, and leaves little room to deviate. It may initially be an adjustment, but think of it as eating the foods you've always been meant to eat.

If you're trying to bring lasting change to your diet, health or even life, maybe Ayurveda is just the thing! Find it an all-encompassing lifestyle program designed to bring real change to every aspect of your life, with solid instructions that have been proved tested and true for centuries.

AYURVEDA ITS RELATIONSHIP WITH FOOD

FOOD TO EAT

In Ayurveda, food is categorized based on physical characteristics and the methods that are said to affect your body. This will help determine the best ingredients for different doshas.

Below are some of the foods you need to eat based on your specific dosha.

PITTA

- Protein: small amounts of chicken, egg white, tofu
- Dairy products: milk, ghee, butter
- Fruits: sweet and ripe fruits such as oranges, pears, pineapples, bananas, melons, mangos
- Vegetables: sweet and bitter vegetables such as cabbage, cauliflower, celery, cucumber, zucchini, leafy vegetables, sweet potato, carrot, squash, brussels sprouts
- Legumes: chickpeas, lentils, mung beans, lima beans, black beans, kidney beans
- Cereals: barley, oats, basmati rice, wheat
- Nuts and seeds: small amounts of pumpkin seeds, flax seeds, sunflower seeds, coconut
- Herbs and spices: small amounts of black husky pepper, cumin, cinnamon, coriander, dill, turmeric

VATA

- Protein: small amounts of chicken, seafood, tofu

- Dairy products: milk, butter, yogurt, cheese, ghee
- Fruits: completely ripe sweet and heavy fruits such as bananas, blueberries, strawberries, grapefruits, mangos, peaches, plums
- Vegetables: cooked vegetables such as beets, sweet potatoes, onions, radishes, turnips, carrots, beans, etc.
- Legumes: chickpeas, lentils, mung beans
- Cereals: cooked oats, cooked rice
- Nuts and seeds: almonds, walnuts, pistachios, chia seeds, flax seeds, sunflower seeds, etc.
- Herbs and spices: cardamom, ginger, cumin, basil, clove, oregano, thyme, black pepper

KAPHA
- Protein: small amounts of poultry, seafood, egg white
- Dairy products: skim milk, goat milk, soy milk
- Fruits: dried fruits such as apples, blueberries, pears, pomegranates, cherries, raisins, figs, prunes
- Vegetables: asparagus, leafy vegetables, onions, potatoes, mushrooms, radish, okra
- Legumes: everything including black beans, chickpeas, lentils, and sponge beans

- Cereals: oats, rye, buckwheat, barley, corn, millet
- Nuts and seeds: small amounts of pumpkin seeds, sunflower seeds, flax seeds
- Herbs and spices: cumin, black hupe pepper, turmeric, raw inger, cinnamon, basil, oregano, thyme, etc.

FOODS TO AVOID

Here are some of the foods that need to be restricted or avoided based on doshas:

PITTA

- Protein: red meat, seafood, egg yolk
- Dairy products: sour cream, cheese, buttermilk
- Fruits: sour or unripe fruits such as grapes, apricots, papayas, grapefruits, sour cherries
- Vegetables: chili, beet, tomato, onion, eggplant
- Cereals: brown rice, millet, corn, rye
- Nuts and seeds: almonds, cashews, peanuts, pine nuts, pistachios, walnuts, sesame
- Herbs and spices: spices not included in the above list

VATA

- Protein: lean meat
- Fruits: dried, immature or light fruits such as raisins, cranberries, pomegranates, pears

- Vegetables: raw vegetables, broccoli, cabbage, cauliflower, mushrooms, potatoes, tomatoes
- Legumes: beans such as black beans, kidney beans, sponge beans
- Cereals: buckwheat, barley, rye, wheat, corn, quinoa, millet
- Herbs and spices: bitter or stringy herbs like parsley, thyme, coriander seeds

KAPHA
- Protein: lean meat, shrimp, egg yolk
- Fruits: banana, coconut, mango, fresh figs
- Vegetables: sweet potato, tomato, zucchini, cucumber
- Legumes: soybeans, kidney beans, taste o
- Cereals: rice, wheat, cooked cereals
- Nuts and seeds: cashew nuts, pecan nuts, pine nuts, Brazil nuts, sesame, walnuts

DOWNSIDES OF AYURVEDA

Although the Ayurvedic diet has several benefits to it, there are drawbacks to consider.

Here are some of the potential Ayurvedic Diet downsides.

One of the major problems with the Ayurvedic diet can be frustrating, because it can be complicated and difficult to follow. There are not only clear lists of foods for each dosha but also a number of additional rules to follow.

For starters, season-based guidelines about which foods you can consume and avoid vary throughout the year. There are also recommendations for when, how often, and how much to eat, which can be challenging — especially for those who are just getting started on the diet.

MAY FEEL OVERLY RESTRICTIVE

There are extensive lists of foods on the Ayurvedic diet which you are advised to eat or avoid depending on your dosha. This can mean cutting off good, whole grains or whole food groups which are believed to aggravate different doshas.

Other ingredients such as red meat or processed foods are also left out which may require significant changes to your current diet. This may feel more rigid and less flexible than other meal plans, and may make it difficult to commit to the long-term diet.

IT IS SUBJECTIVE

Another problem with the Ayurvedic diet is the subjectivity of it.

The diet focuses on determining your dominant dosha which is based on a set of physical and mental characteristics.

While there are plenty of tips and online quizzes available to help ease the process, it isn't foolproof to find out the dosha.

As the diet guidelines are specific to each dosha, choosing the wrong dosha could have an adverse effect on your performance.

In addition, there is currently no evidence supporting the concept of doshas or the claim that your personality traits determine what foods you should eat and avoid. So it's unknown how effective the diet is, even if you decide the dosha correctly.

PRINCIPLES & PRACTICES OF AYURVEDA

Ayurveda is India's traditional medical method, which literally translated means "study or knowledge of life" Its origin dates back an estimated 5-10,000 years, and is widely regarded as the world's oldest form of health care. Many historians agree that it inspired the ancient Chinese philosophy of medicine, Unani medicine, and the humoral medicine studied by Hippocrates in Greece as understanding of Ayurveda spread out from India.

Because of this, Ayurveda is often referred to as the "Mother of All Healing." Ayurveda knowledge has its written origins in the Vedas, India's sacred texts, believed to be the world's oldest writings. The Vedas, written in Sanskrit, cover a large number of topics, from grammar to health care. The Vedas were written about or earlier than 2500BC.

Most of the current knowledge about Ayurveda derives from comparatively later writings, mainly the Caraka Samhita (around 1500 BC), the Ashtang Hrdyam (around 500 AD), and the Sushrut Samhita (around 300-400 AD). These three classics describe the basic principles and theories Ayurveda developed from. We also provide extensive scientific knowledge on treating a variety of diseases. Later writings and research expand on this early information about clinics.

Ayurveda is based on the premise that illness is the natural end result of living in harmony with our surroundings. Natural is an important word, since Ayurveda recognizes that sickness signs are the normal way in which the body expresses disharmony. With this understanding of illness, Ayurveda's healing approach becomes evident: to restore harmony between self and environment.

When recovered, the body's need to express disharmony reduces, symptoms dissipate, and cure is said to have happened.
Ayurveda understands every person and the illness that the person manifests as a unique entity. No two people are alike and no two diseases are alike, it could be said. Consequently, Ayurveda does not approach the cure of an illness as much as it approaches a person's cure.

This approach differs vastly from allopathic medicine. Where allopathic medicine seeks a drug that will cure for a specific condition a statistically significant number of people, such as rheumatoid arthritis, Ayurvedic medicine seeks a treatment that will cure an individual person from their unique presentation of the disease. Since no illness affects two people exactly the same way, there are no two cures that are exactly the same.

PRINCIPLES

For the Ayurvedic practitioner, the nature of the patient, the nature of the disease, and the nature of the remedy need to be understood. Only then can a doctor provide the best attention. Nature's qualities are said to be heavy or light, cold or hot, stable or mobile, sharp or sluggish, moist or dry, subtle or gross, dense or flowing, soft or hard, smooth or raw or cloudy or clear.

It is understood that a person, a disease or a remedy has a unique combination of these qualities. The aim of the Ayurvedic practitioner is to understand as many of the qualities as possible regarding their patient and the condition of their patient.
A person may be heavy or light, may move quickly or slowly, may feel warmer or cooler, may have a sharp or slender mind, may have moist or dry skin. These are examples of an understanding of a person's nature.

Likewise, a disease such as arthritis can be characterized as causing severe or dull pain, migrating (mobile) or localizing into one or more joints (stable), inducing vasodilatation around the joint (warm), or vascular constriction (cool). The nature of a condition is recognized by recognizing the appearance of a disorder through its characteristics.

Herbal remedies are also known according to their consistency. Nourishing things, such as licorice, are described as hard. The depleting compounds are colored, for example red clover. Many plants, such as ginger, produce fire in the body and others cool the body, such as goldenseal. Throughout Ayurveda, the fundamental principle of diagnosis is the management of the illness with characteristics opposite to its existence. Cold diseases are treated with mild remedies, light treatments are used to treat serious diseases, and so on.

Ayurveda describes the human being as being composed of 5 elements, 3 doshas (biological energies), 7 dhatus (tissues), and numerous srotas (channels). The five elements are ether, air, fire, water, earth and land. These five elements, which also constitute all of Nature, are not intended to be taken literally. Those are ideas that are described as elements.

They are the respective ideas of space, motion, heat, flow, and solidity. We have the aforementioned characteristics. These elements are composed of the three doshas, the biological forces which govern the functions of the body.

Vata dosha is a biological force that governs every movement in the body. It's made up of ether and air and is light, warm, mobile and cool. Individuals with this force predominating in their bodies tend to exhibit these traits. They seem to be thin, they have dry skin, they feel cold quickly, they walk and they talk easy. They also tend to have a larger amount of cold emotion, such as fear and anxiety.

Vata dosha deficiency can affect any body system, and may lead to an increase in these qualities. For example, as seen in dry asthma and non-productive coughs the respiratory system becomes dry. The digestive system gets dry and constipated, an irregular activity.

Dryness may precipitate stone formation in the kidneys or gall bladder and hyper-excitability is known to cause an increase in the mobile content of vata in the nervous system. Vata's cold disposition can get seriously disturbed and trigger Raynaud's Phenomenon. Wasting conditions are seen as an improvement in the quality of light from vata.

Therefore there will be physiological disturbance wherever in the body there is an increase in the qualities of vata.

Pitta dosha is a force that regulates all digestion in the body. Composed mainly of fire, flow is hot, light, sharp, and exhibits. It contains a small amount of water, and is therefore neither very moist nor dry.

Those qualities are exhibited by people with predominance of pitta in their bodies. They feel warm and have less of a cold weather effect. They have a rosy complexion, are moderate in weight and reasonably steady, build a mesomorphic body and can have a sharp and intense personality. A greater amount of intense feelings, such as anger, bitterness, and envy, continue to contradict this trait.

The digestive system appears to be powerful, since pitta controls digestion. Digestion of food is a small problem. Bowel movements frequently occur, 2-3X per day.

Pitta dosha deficiency can affect any system in the body but is predisposed to affect a lot of fire-containing systems. When pitta affects a system, at that location generally greater heat builds. Liver, small intestine, blood, skin, and eyes are systems that exert great influence on pitta.

Examples of heated pitta conditions in those body regions are hepatitis, hyperacidity, acne, and conjunctivitis. Pitta disruption can affect any system. Infections which produce heat and fever anywhere in the body are known as pitta disorders.

Kapha dosha is a biological force that governs organic growth. It is heavy, moist, stable, soft, and dull composed of water and earth. Individuals with kapha predominance in their bodies tend to weigh more, have heavier, denser bones and skin, and build a more typical endomorphic body. You do tend to have smooth moist skin, and long, full hair.

Personality of that person tends to be relaxed and not easily disturbed. They are listening, just moving slowly. The heavy feelings, such as lethargy and rigidity, can challenge them. When kapha grows in the body, there is a greater production of mucous that is heavy, thick, and moist like kapha.

Swelling, and weight gain can also occur. While kapha can affect any body system, the most vulnerable are the stomach and the lungs. This is where we see several common kapha disturbance signs— nausea, limited appetite, and mucous formation. Conditions like obesity, some cancers, chronic bronchitis, lung congestion and syndromes of fluid retention have kapha disorder as a component of pathophysiology.

While the doshas are seen as the causative agents of the disease, the source of the disease is known as dhatus, upadhatus, and srotas. Dhatus is tissue, upadhatus is extra tissue and srotas are channel structures. Seven tissues are present; serum, blood, muscle, skin, bone, marrow, and reproductive tissue.

Unlike Western medicine, which understands that each tissue is different, Ayurveda understands that each is dependent for its nutrition and health on the tissues which precede it. Consequently, a disease that arises in one area can inevitably have global implications if not fixed.

Pathology in Ayurveda in terms of what dosha influences what dhatu can be partly understood. This dhatu is smaller, drier, and hyper-mobile as vata reaches a dhatu. It gets heated when pitta enters and when kapha enters it becomes heavier, moister, and more stable. In a muscle, vata disruption causes wasting and atrophy, infection and inflammation causes pitta disturbance, and premature development causes kapha disturbance.

Srotas are close communication systems to the human body's organ systems. The major srotas are somewhat equivalent to the respiratory, digestive, reproductive, cardiovascular, urinary, and water metabolism system. These are alternate disease sites where doshas can get worse.

Ayurveda accepts that metabolic waste is created during the body's metabolic processes and has to be carefully removed to preserve optimum health. Products from the waste are called malas. Another causative cause in disability is the disruption of their removal.

-individual has a constitution, as defined at birth, according to Ayurveda. The underlying equilibrium of these three doshas is this Constitution. The Constitution establishes the basic form and temperament of a person's body. While other factors influence body and personality development, the constitution provides the predisposition in much the same way as the biology of an individual.

Ayurveda is a common misconception of grouping people according to three forms. Actually there are infinite combinations and permutations in each individual of these three fundamental energies. Hence we see that it is known that each individual is special.

The first goal of the Ayurvedic practicer is to consider the patient's condition or structure. It shows the doctor who it is that they handle.
Next the doctor tries to understand either the disorder or the essence of the difference. Ayurvedic disease is understood in terms of dosing imbalance and attributes imbalance within the body.

The practicer tests the body's doshas, dhatus, upadhatus, srotas, and malas. The overall strength of the body is and is also being measured as an important factor in potential care. The term ojas is applied to the resilience of the muscle, though it is more precisely the one that gives the body the ability to withstand pain.

Although pathology is essential to understand the origin of the disease, etiology is equally important. Etiology is understood according to how the diet, behaviors and climate of the individual induced disruption of the doshas. A lifestyle that stresses rapid pace, work or relationship shifts, travel, fast foods, and fresh, light foods— such as a vegetarian diet— is likely to cause vata dosha aggravation.

Pitta is likely to worsen a lifestyle that is stressful, aggressive, highly focused, and that stresses spicy hot foods. Kapha is aggravated by a sedentary lifestyle and a diet of strong, fatty foods, including milk, yogurt, and beef.

THERAPY TYPES

The therapist can now devise a treatment program to bring the patient back into balance, recognizing the essence of the client and the complexity of the condition. The program uses as its basis what is commonly called five sense therapy, together with advanced mind and body purification and rejuvenation procedures.
Using the sense of taste, the doctor may administer a diet which consists of the disease's opposite quality or imbalance.

This diet is very specific and it describes the exact foods a patient may consume in each category. That includes meats, dairy, nuts, vegetables, etc. The practitioner also recommends herbs that work in accordance with similar principles. Ayurveda recognizes, in addition to the effects that herbs have on the body's energies and qualities, that some herbs also have the ability to have strong effects on specific organs and symptoms. In formulations creation this assumption is taken into account.

Color therapies are used using the sense of vision. Colors are known to have the same qualities as all of Nature and, again, colors are recommended which have the disease's opposite qualities. When developing a medication, colours can have significant special effects on specific diseases, and this is understood and considered.

The lungs use hearing therapy to provide a platform for diagnosis. Ayurveda has historically used sound vibrations for healing, or mantras. Various sounds have different effects on the dosha. Such sound energies are known to activate different organs and endocrine glands which may influence the development of hormones.

Aroma therapy includes diagnosis through sense of smell. The properties of an odor have different effects on the doshas. Sweet-smelling fragrances, for example, boost kapha but bring balance to vata and pitta.

The application of specific oils and massage is utilized through the skin. Different stresses and pressures have different effects on doshas. The patient may be told to apply massage to itself, or the practitioner may apply the massage.

Ayurveda merges with its Indian sister science for the treatment of the mind: yoga. The patient is encouraged to adopt a lifestyle that emphasizes peace of mind and connection to God through yoga and meditation. The consequent elimination of tension is an accepted part of the healing process.

Ayurveda also stresses the importance of keeping your body pure and clean. Toxins, both external and intrinsic to the body, interfere with the flow of waste material from the cells which leads to impaired function. Ayurveda employs a technique known as Panchakarma, meaning "the five actions," to remove these toxins.

This is a program performed at a specialized center for 7-28 days. Panchakarma uses a restricted diet, acupuncture therapy, extra medicated oil treatments, medicated vapor therapies and detox therapies such as enemas, purgation, and nasal /

sinus cleaning of special oils snorted into the nasal passages. That last therapy is called nasya.

Historically, and nowadays in some parts of the world, two extra treatments are used. We are medicinal diarrhea and leeches releasing milk. The patient withdraws from the world in addition to these physical modalities and enjoys time for meditation and reflection.

While each therapy is understood to be important, Ayurveda emphasizes analysis and change of lifestyle as the most important aspect of the healing process. The practitioner helps a patient understand how lifestyle has contributed to the origin of the present condition and provides support as the patient attempts to create a new lifestyle more in keeping with their constitution.

After assessing the patient, the Ayurvedic practitioner designs a program that uses the above mentioned therapies. These therapies can be instituted over a period of time and are not generally prescribed all at once, as they can prove overwhelming for a patient to successfully implement.

Demographics There are no systematic surveys of how many patients and their lives are using Ayurvedic treatment and concepts. As Ayurveda in the West is a relatively new science, the percentage is likely to be low. Worldwide, Ayurveda's traditional medicine is still used primarily by the Indian poor, who can not afford Western medicine.

Referral Ayurveda indications and reasons is a complete medical science that should be considered when allopathic medicine can not produce the desired results. Given that Ayurveda provides guidelines for the treatment of every body system, it can play a role in any case management. It is most effectively used on chronic and sub-acute disease patients in the United States. Acute conditions are usually not advised. Ayurvedic lifestyle treatments can also be successfully used to improve health and reduce sickness.

Science Foundation Work in Ayurveda has focused on the use of Indian herbs in pharmacology. Literature describing medicinal components, acts, signs, and contraindications is plentiful in the journals of botanical and Ayurvedic medicine. Successful therapies are well known for a multitude of natural herbal diseases from India. Clinical evidence shows that Ayurvedic therapy has few harmful side effects, and this is backed by anecdotal evidence for 5000 years.

DRUG-LIKE INFORMATION AND SAFETY
The actions of most herbs have not been studied in great detail and the cross-reactions of herbs and drugs. History suggests few adverse experiences, and in a trained practitioner's hands most herbs are healthy. Practitioners are informed about which woman pregnant and lactating should stop medicines and procedures.

Botanical research journals contain the latest information about many herbs ' actions, effects, and side effects. Nadkarni's Indian Materia Medica is the main book that summarizes herbal research used in Ayurveda.

VISITING A PROFESSIONAL
A patient visiting an Ayurvedic practitioner should expect to receive an assessment consisting of: a minimum of a history of the chief complaint, past medical history, system review, and a review of any medication— such as herbs and vitamins that the patient may take.

Observations are made of face shape, neck size, eye size and depth, hair colour, quantity and quality, skin thickness and bone width. Detailed test procedures include pulse and language. Examination of the belly and recording vital signs completes the examination.

The doctor spends time telling the patient on their results after the test, which usually lasts for one hour or more. The practitioner educates the patient about Ayurveda and its imbalances during the course of this findings report. To Ayurveda it is said that what the patient knows is more important than what the practitioner knows.

A patient should be going back to health with a clear understanding of their path. Follow-up visits are planned to support patients as they advance and confront challenges. Follow-up tours include ongoing counselling and training. Over time, additional therapies are slowly integrated into the program, as the patient strives to create a lifestyle of harmony through the five senses.

CREDENTIALING AND TRAINING
There are currently only a few places in the U.S. where the practitioners receive thorough training. The duration of programs varies from one to two years, and often involves part-time classroom and independent study. Graduates of the California

College of Ayurveda in California receive certification as a "Clinical Ayurvedic Specialist" and use the initials C.A.S.

This is the only institution in the United States that offers the practitioner complete clinical training. Many curricula differ in length and concentration. At most schools the emphasis is on Ayurveda's metaphysical and fundamental concepts. There are also home-study classes offered by the American Vedic Studies Institute and by unique instructors. Some services also focus on the values of theory and fundamentals.

When searching for an Ayurveda practitioner, evaluate the extent of their education. Check to see if anybody or any agency has approved their certification. When appropriate, investigate the certifying agency. Seek to always visit the doctor and discuss the cases they've handled and their outcomes. Question how they handle cases, and which measures they use to assess development. Ayurveda California College maintains a list of graduate practitioners across the USA.

HOW TO TRANSFORM YOUR RELATIONSHIP WITH FOOD USING AYURVEDIC

Ayurvedic Medicine" may sound like something technical or complicated but it's far from it. This practice, commonly referred to as "Ayurveda," is an ancient practice of holistic medicine rooted in India thousands of years ago. Despite its age and reputation around the world, in recent years it has only begun to make its way to Western kitchens. Emphasizing the body-mind link, Ayurveda is not about curing sickness, but rather about encouraging life-long wellbeing through positive lifestyle habits.

Ayurveda, as a holistic philosophy, accepts multiple facets of one's life— sleep, pain, mindfulness, and, of course, diet. And no, we don't say "diet" in the sense of losing weight and taking off food groups, but rather the mindset that food has the amazing ability to feed our body and soul when eaten properly.

While modern fad diets due to their restrictive nature can lead to a negative relationship with food, Ayurveda celebrates the medicinal aspect of food, and the incredible ability of the body to transform food into nutrients and energy. Moreover, Ayurveda emphasizes establishing a positive relationship with food, with simple mantras that can be applied to any lifestyle or cooking.

Those who follow Ayurveda believe digestion is at the heart of good health. What good are the nutrients in our food, after all, if our body can't absorb them properly? That's why it's not just about what we eat but also about how we eat. Here are a few simple ways to integrate Ayurveda into your daily routine.

Sit Down and Slow Down at Meal Time With the busy lives we all live, meal time seems to have lost its place, as people opt for grab-n-go meals and lunches at the desk. Nevertheless, slowly taking the time to sit down and enjoy your food is vital, because when we rush through the meals we end up not thoroughly chewing food, which impedes proper digestion. Take this as an opportunity to relax and enjoy the flavors of your meal in full.

Eat The Main Meal of the Day at Lunch According to Ayurvedic medicine, do like the Spaniards and eat the biggest meal at midday (not at night). Perhaps the most important component of ayurvedic diet is the idea of feeding when one's digestive capacity becomes best. Because one's agni, or "digestive gas," is at its highest mid-day capacity, this allows the body to thoroughly digest a big lunch until evening, when digestion begins to close.

Despite the temptation to catch up on social media while munching, watching screens activates our central nervous system that may interfere with digestion. Worse still, the screens prevent us from paying full attention to what's on our plate, which can lead to overeating. Instagram can wait; let your food stand in the spotlight for its moment.

Consider Organic, Whole Foods Your Best Friends An important principle in Ayurveda is that in order to achieve good health our lives and bodies should be in accordance with the earth. One principal reason for this is that our bodies have the inherent ability to process the most natural foods. Therefore make sure that natural, healthy foods are at the center of your diet, and keep clear of processed foods and foods with artificial or preservative additives. If you are focusing colorfully on food, you're on the right track already.

Stay Hydrated, But Ditch the Ice Water You know the importance of staying hydrated already. What you may not have known is that water at warm or room temperature is actually much better for digestion, particularly right before or after a meal. The body must do much more to digest cold water and this cycle hinders digestion by reducing blood flow and digestive enzyme activity.

Nevertheless, warm water is easily digested and also helps in nutrient absorption. Throughout the day and at meals, sipping warm water will not only keep you hydrated but also help you get faster.

Being Spice-Friendly Spices is an essential part of having Ayurvedic food. Spices, the ultimate multitaskers, add immense flavor to food, while boosting natural immunity and kicking digestion in gear. Take your cooking to the next level by throwing cumin, ginger, turmeric and coriander in some of the classic Ayurvedic spices.

In addition, the use of spices will help you to incorporate all six flavors: sweet, sour, salty, bitter, astringent and pungent, which is another important element of Ayurvedic cooking.

Allow After Meals Downtime Whether it's reading, going for a walk, or even meditating if that's your thing, you should always take the time to relax after a meal before moving on with your day. This isn't to suggest that when you finish grubbing you should become a couch potato (lying down after a meal will potentially impede digestion), so allowing yourself a transition period before jumping right into the next task allows for optimum digestion.

If you're able to embrace these simple Ayurvedic mantras, you're going to master your mindful eating and enhancing your food relationship (while boosting your mental and physical health).

CHAPTER TWO

AYURVEDIC CARE FOR RHEUMATOID ARTHRITIS:

What to know Many Ayurvedic physicians use Ayurveda to cure rheumatoid arthritis (RA), which they call amavata. Ayurvedic treatment may include vitamins, dietary changes, and exercise.

Here we review Ayurvedic RA treatment, including the basic principles, and whether it is supported by research.

GENERAL PRINCIPLES
The word "Ayurveda" is a mixture of the words "ayu" (life) and "veda" (knowledge) in Sanskrit. Practitioners work to balance life's three energy forces, or "doshas,": "vata," "pitta," and "kapha." Ayurvedic RA treatments depend on what diagnostic guidelines the practitioner uses.

For example, those who practice from the "Madhava Nidana" guidelines believe imbalances in the intestines and inflammatory compounds cause RA.

On the other hand, "Ashtanga Hridaya" school of thought practitioners believe that RA is the result of poor dietary and lifestyle habits which cause inflammation in the body.

Both approaches use herbs, supplements, changes in diet and exercise to help alleviate RA symptoms. The practice of Ayurvedic herbs and supplements often involves the use of herbs and supplements as treatment.

Some of the herbs that Ayurvedic practitioners often use to treat RA include: • Boswellia serrata (Indian frankincense) • garlic• ginger • Ricinus communis (castor oil) • ashwagandha Some formulations of Ayurvedic medicine also contain bhasma, which are specially prepared forms of metals such as silver, copper and iron.

An Ayurvedic practitioner may also prepare special medicinal oils. Individuals will rub these oils into places where symptoms arise.
Ayurvedic drugs are not regulated by the Food and Drug Administration (FDA) in the same manner as prescription medicines.
As a result, there is less research on how supplements function, how they may interfere with

other prescription medicines, and if they are healthy.

It is therefore vital that individuals only buy Ayurvedic supplements from a reputable practitioner and tell their doctor if they are using Ayurvedic treatments.

We should also ask their Ayurvedic doctor precisely what's in each preparation and make sure it doesn't contain any chemicals that a person is allergic to or can interfere with other medical treatments.

Diet Ayurvedic practitioners believe that the following dietary habits can cause or worsen RA symptoms: • drinking alcohol•eating spicy foods • eating excess salt • eating too many sour, sweet, or sugar foods• eating uncooked foods• eating acid reflux foods As a result, an Ayurvedic practitioner will recommend avoiding these foods.

Some Ayurvedic practitioners also recommend barley and rice soups, as they are thought to add a sense of lightness to the body.

A doctor may sometimes easily prescribe a castor oil. This is when a person consumes castor oil, a natural laxative, to facilitate intestinal cleansing.

A person will reintroduce foods over several days, and ultimately advance to a healthy routine diet.

Ayurvedic practitioners think positive lifestyle habits can support RA treatment.
We claim a sedentary lifestyle leads to "ama" being created, causing inflammation and disease.

Practicing yoga, an essential component of ayurvedic medicine, can help a person with RA become more involved and relieve stiffness and discomfort, too.
Ayurvedic practitioners may recommend the following tips for people with RA:

- to use hot water, not cold, to bathe and drink
- to avoid exposure to cold breezes
- to avoid late-night or late-afternoon naps • to practice yoga to relieve mental stress
- to use herbal oils massage therapy to reduce pain and stiffness While Ayurvedic practitioners believe that physical activity can help relieve mental stress.

What's the Report saying?

There is little comprehensive and recent work directly on Ayurvedic therapies for RA. Researchers report difficulties in designing clinical trials to test Ayurvedic interventions, compared to modern medicine or placebos. Many studies are small, making it hard for researchers to know whether the results would be applicable to larger populations.

A study published in the International Journal of Ayurveda Research in 2011 for example studied ayurvedic therapies in 290 people with RA over 7 years.
At the conclusion of the study, the author found that improvements were reported by even participants with severe RA including reductions in swelling and pain. The study did not use a control group though, so the results are hard to confirm.

Other, lesser case studies support the use of Ayurveda in the treatment of RA individuals. The use of Ayurveda to alleviate RA symptoms was confirmed by a 2015 case report on Ayurvedic therapy in a 45-year-old female. The therapy included acupuncture, vitamins, a strong castor oil, avoiding spicy foods, and eating foods "sweet."

In contemporary research, some aspects of ayurvedic treatment are given more support. Many Ayurvedic practitioners for example recommend yoga to help relieve symptoms of RA.

A 2018 study of 75 RA adults found that yoga improved fitness, flexibility, mood, and overall quality of life related to health.

Overview Sadly there is little work of high quality to justify the use of Ayurvedic RA therapies.

However, many of the dietary and exercise-related changes may be beneficial, with the supervision of a doctor. Any reduced inflammation is also expected to be helpful. Because RA can damage joints without effective treatment, it is important to work with an Ayurvedic practitioner together with a rheumatology doctor.

There is currently no licensing scheme in the United States for Ayurvedic practitioners nor is there a formal training or certification process. That is different from India's Ayurvedic training, which has many regulations.

Anyone considering ayurvedic treatment should speak with their regular physician and be sure to ask about the training and safety practices of an ayurvedic practitioner.

AYURVEDA AND PSORIASIS

Psoriasis is an inflammatory condition which affects the skin, causing skin cells to grow excessively and rapidly. This can lead to thick, scaly plaques forming.

Ayurvedic medicine includes ingredients which have also been used by other medical disciplines to treat psoriasis, such as aloe vera and turmeric.

While in some people Ayurveda may be able to treat psoriasis, researchers declined to perform large-scale clinical trials and systematic reviews to determine its safety and effectiveness.

Here we look at Ayurveda's benefits to people with psoriasis. We are also reviewing the study into whether it delivers effective treatment.

A person with psoriasis on their skin could use Ayurvedic preparations.

In Ayurvedic medicine one of the most common topical preparations contains turmeric. Manufacturers produce the turmeric from a ginger-like plant root.

Typically Turmeric appears in cooking. People can mix it into a paste, however, and apply it to the skin too.

Meditation and activity Ayurvedic teachings promote a harmony of three "elements," which they describe as: • the world of an individual• the structure of the body, or "Prakriti"• the essential powers of the body, or "dosha" One way a person should hold these in check is by minimizing stress and anxiety.

Meditation and the practice of "Pranayama," a controlled technique of breathing, may benefit a person in reducing their psoriasis.
Such methods of mindfulness may help the overall wellbeing of a person. As stress is a potential trigger for psoriasis flares, these relaxation techniques could help prevent a flare by reducing stress levels.
Dietary changes Typically Ayurvedic practices revolve around a vegetarian diet. High-carbohydrate ingredients and products containing large amounts of sugar are also foods to avoid.

Ayurvedic practices also suggest that a person should avoid "extreme" foods, such as tastes that are too salty, too sour or too acidic.
Practitioners in Ayurveda recommend that a person "listen" to his body. For example, they clear their body of toxins by responding to urinating or defecating urges.

While dietary changes can not specifically cure psoriasis, the University of California-San Francisco School of Medicine's (UCSF) Department of Dermatology conducted a survey of dietary habits for people with psoriasis.

The results suggested that people with advanced diets, such as a vegan, and paleo or high-protein and low-carb diet, have seen symptom changes. This statement reflects the idea that Ayurvedic dietary choices are healthy for people with psoriasis.

Topical solutions A lot of other Ayurvedic compounds and herbs are available, as well as turmeric, and several could potentially benefit people with psoriasis.
People who have used ayurvedic herbs to treat psoriasis include:

- Aloe vera
- Black nightshade
- Boswellia, or frankincense
- Garlic
- Guggul
- Jasmine flower paste
- Neem

The National Psoriasis Foundation recommends topical aloe vera to soothing itchy skin. We encourage people to select creams with an aloe content of 0.5 per cent.

The efficacy of other therapies is backed only by anecdotal evidence.

Although they may promote overall health, no research supports their use as psoriasis treatments. However, if they provide relief and after using them people don't experience side effects, they are safe to try. A person with psoriasis can consider using these therapies, alongside scientifically supported medications, as complementary.

People should ask advice from their doctor before adding Ayurvedic medicines into their routine.

Having regular baths helps keep areas of psoriasis lesions soft and clean. In addition, baths can be soothing and reduce stress, which may offer additional benefits in reducing the incidence of flares from psoriasis.

The application of natural soothing oils, such as coconut or olive oils, can help soften the skin and relieve the psoriasis itching and discomfort.

How Ayurveda explains psoriasis According to Ayurvedic research practitioners, psoriasis is classified as a "kushtha" state of health. The term means that "krucchasadhya," meaning intractable, and "asadhya," meaning incurable is a chronic condition.

Ayurvedic texts say the psoriasis is caused by an excess between two "doshas," or energy fields. Ayurvedic medicine traditions call both "Vata" and "Kapha." Vata is responsible for controlling body functions, and may lead to psoriasis dryness and skin scaling. Kapha is responsible for growth, so the Ayurvedic practitioners use this dosha to understand the itching and rapid skin cell turnover.

The disparity between these two forces allows toxins to build up, leading to inflammation, in a person's system. Consequently, Ayurvedic therapies also revolve around not only herbal formulations but also guidance on diet and lifestyle.
Study
There are many Ayurvedic therapies but small scale and often observational trials. Nonetheless, the effect of some common Ayurvedic therapies on psoriatic skin lesions has been tested by researchers.

Several studies suggest that psoriasis involvement in the skin may be reduced by ayurvedic treatment.

A study published in the Iranian Journal of Pharmaceutical Research in 2015 reported the effects of turmeric gel on a group of people with moderate to mild psoriasis.

After nine weeks, the researchers assessed the participants for skin redness, lesion thickness and lesion size.

The researchers discovered that those who applied the turmeric gel experienced less redness, thickness and scaling than those who applied placebo.

The authors of the study have also confirmed that the application of the gel had few side effects.

A different study in the journal Clinical Dermatology found that topical applications of 3-O-Acetyl-11 Keto Beta Boswellic Acid (AKBBA) helped manage chronic plaque psoriasis, which is mild to moderate.

AKBBA is a gum resin naturally occurring from the Boswellia serrate tree stem.

Over 12 weeks, individuals with psoriasis started applying the cream three times a day. Scientists checked photos after the 12-week duration to identify any improvements in lesions caused by psoriasis. The leaders of the study reported highly significant lesion improvements, and proposed AKBBA as a possible treatment for psoriasis.

In treating psoriasis, a 2015 study reported the effects of a starch fortified turmeric bath (SFTB), a mixture of rice starch and turmeric.
A control group took part in therapies including massage, yoga, hydrotherapy, and diet therapy. The experimental group used both these and the SFTB therapies.
The researchers found that SFTBs decreased both the severity of psoriasis and the spread of lesions. They concluded that SFTBs may be a complementary low-cost therapy in psoriasis management.

Risks and safety considerations Ayurveda has been around for thousands of years, as a medical practice. Research which supports or disputes its claims, however, is not widely available.
Most Ayurveda studies are small, and they do not use the type of research methods that support firm conclusions.

Therefore it is difficult to say with great certainty that Ayurveda can help to reduce the frequency of outbreaks of psoriasis or their physical effects. Yet many people report that they have been improved by Ayurveda.

Ayurvedic products are currently classified as dietary supplements by the United States Food and Drug Administration (FDA). This ensures they don't have to go through the same rigorous testing of safety and efficacy as many other drugs.

Some Ayurvedic products are advised by the National Center for Complementary and Integrative Health to contain unsafe levels of lead, mercury and arsenic that may be toxic.

Consumers should be careful when using Ayurvedic products, even if they are marked as' all-natural' by the manufacturers. People should not use Ayurvedic products as a substitute for other medical treatments unless they discuss this with their doctor.

Summary Ayurveda is an ancient medical practice but there is limited research into its safety and efficacy.

In the management of psoriasis some herbs and organic products, such as turmeric and aloe vera, are already common.

Meditation and yoga practices that accompany Ayurveda may also help people with psoriasis support their well-being and psychological health, but scientific evidence of Ayurveda's positive effects on psoriatic skin is minimal or too small for wider use.

If the effects of psoriasis are moderate to severe, or fail to respond to alternative therapies, patients may consider other choices with their doctor.

CHAPTER THREE
BEVERAGES AND BREAKFASTS

VATA BEVERAGES AND BREAKFAST

CINNAMON HONEY MILK SHAKE

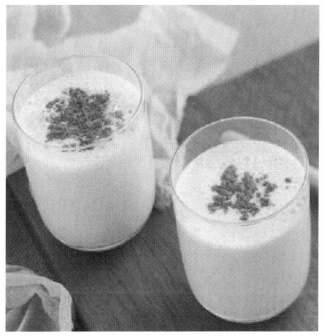

INGREDIENTS
- Eggs, 2
- dried Honey

- 5 teaspoon Ginger
- 1/4 teaspoons, freshly ground Cinnamon
- 1/4 teaspoons, ground Ghee,
- 1 tablespoon Whole Organic Dairy, 8 oz.

PREPARATIONS

Step 1: If your dates already include holes, cut them by chopping one side down.

Step 2: Warm the 8 ounces of milk in the microwave for 30 seconds.

Step 3: Dump each ingredient into your blender. Mix until distilled.

Step 4: Serve in a warm travel mug and enjoy.

SPICED WARM MILK

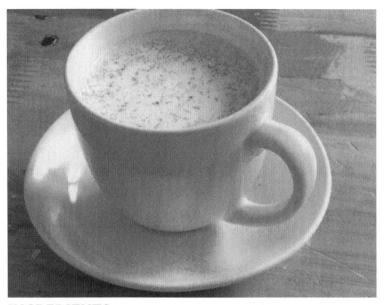

INGREDIENTS
- Whole Organic Milk, 8 ounces
- Cinnamon, small pinch (optional)
- Dry Ginger, small pinch (optional)

PREPARATIONS

Step 1: Pour your organic milk into a microwave safe drinking mug

Step 2: Add the above-mentioned warm spices if you like. It's Stir.

Step 3: 20-30 seconds of microwave. Based on the strength of your microwave, the cooking time may be significantly shorter or longer than 20-30 seconds.
Step 4: Mix again to make sure the spices are mixed.
Step 5: Love it!

WARMING OATMEAL

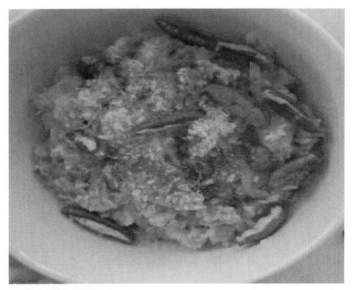

INGREDIENTS
- Sliced almonds
- 2 teaspoons Sugar
- 1 teaspoon Cinnamon
- 1/4 teaspoons Cardamom
- 1/4 teaspoons Ghee

- 1 teaspoon Prunes
- 3 dried apricots
- 3 dry sugar
- 1/2 teaspoon Himalayan salt
- pinch Ginger
- 1 tablespoon, raw, grated Oats,

PREPARATIONS

Step 1: Soak almonds and dried fruit in water overnight

Step 2: Position water, berries, grated gypsum, bring this mixture to a boil.

Step 3: When the water boils, add the oats. Switch the flame off, so the oatmeal is just simmering. Usually, this is low. Stir the oatmeal regularly and simmer for 10 minutes.

Step 4: When the 10-minute mark is reached, remove the oatmeal from the stove, stir again and cover. Let this sit down for about two minutes.

Step 5: Now incorporate the remaining ingredients (ghee, herbs, tea, nuts). Stir well, serve soft.

PITTA BEVERAGES AND BREAKFAST

POMEGRANATE ALOE DRINK

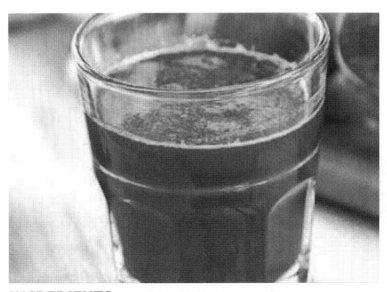

INGREDIENTS
- Turbinado Sugar
- 2 teaspoons Pomegranate Juice
- 1 cup Lime
- 1, fresh Aloe Vera
- 1 tablespoon, Gel

PREPARATIONS
Step 1: Lime juice.
Step 2: Combine the other ingredients, stirring until the sugar is mostly dissolved.

Step 3: Serve in a chilled glass with a slice of lime to garnish.

REJUVENATING BANANA SMOOTHIE

INGREDIENTS
- Lime
- 5 fresh Coconut Water
- 1 cup Cardamom
- 2 Fresh Banana

PREPARATION
Step 1: Juice half a lime and add juice to the blender. Scrape any remaining pulp in the peel for added flavor.
Step 2: Put the remaining ingredients in the blender. Puree until it's clean.
Step 3: Serve in a chilled glass, finished with a basil leaf.

WAFFLES-PUMPKIN SPICE, TOPPED WITH NUTTY-MAPLE SYRUP.

INGREDIENTS
- Spelt Flour

- 1 teaspoon Himalayan Salt
- Pinch Turbinado Sugar
- 1 tablespoon Pumpkin
- 5 cups, canned or pre-baked* Ghee
- 5 pieces Eggs
- 3 cups Powder
- 1 tablespoon Almond Milk
- 1 cup Pecans
- 1 tablespoon Maple Syrup
- 1/4 teaspoon Himalayan salt pinch

PREPARATIONS

To prepare the waffle topping:

Step 1: pour the pecans into a pan over high heat and toast.

Step 2: Break the pecans into small pieces.

Step3: Combine maple syrup, chopped pecans and a pinch of salt in a small dish.

PUMPKIN

Step 1: In a small pan, melt the ghee on a low heat burner. Set it to the side.

Step 2: Mix the baking powder, starch, sugar and salt in a small mixing bowl.

Step 3: Using a small mixing dish, beat the pumpkin, the eggs and the ghee with a whisk.

Step 4: Put the cooked batter in a pre-fatand pre-heated waffle iron. Check the owner's manual for recommended amounts, as each iron is special.
Step 5: Remove from the iron the cooked waffles.
Phase 6: Serve soft with Nutty-Maple Syrup.

KAPHA BEVERAGES AND BREAKFAST

WATERMELON SMOOTHIE LEMON

INGREDIENTS
- 2 Wedges Lime
- New Cardamom 1/5 Teaspoons, Ground
- New Watermelon 2 Cups, In Cubes

PREPARATIONS
Step 1: Extract all the seeds from the watermelon parts.
Phase 2: Put the dried watermelon in a blender. Squeeze the wedges of lime over the watermelon. Sprinkle with cardamom over the top. Puree until it's smooth.

Step 3: Serve in a chilled glass, garnish with a lime slice.

UPGRADED GRAPEFRUIT

INGREDIENTS
- Honey, 1 teaspoon
- Raw grapefruit
- 1, fresh ginger
- 1/4 teaspoons, ground cardamom
- 1/4 teaspoons, dried cardamom (optional)

PREPARATIONS
Step 1: In a small bowl, combine honey, cardamom and ginger.
Step 2: Break off the top and bottom of your grapefruit.
Step 3: Place the grapefruit on one of these now smooth sides and, starting at the top, split it between the rind and the skin, following the curve of the fruit.
Step 4: First, cut the insides of the membrane partitions and extract the slice. Repeat until all the slices are clear from grapefruit.
Step 5: Put all slices of grapefruit in a bowl containing honey and spices. Enjoy your delicious breakfast.

IMMUNE BOOSTING MILK

INGREDIENTS
- Turmeric
- 1/4 teaspoons Milk
- 1 cup Honey
- 1 teaspoon Cinnamon
- 1/4 teaspoon Cardamom

PREPARATIONS

Step 1: Place milk, cardamom, cinnamon and turmeric in a small saucepan. Stir constantly, flame until it melts.

Step 2: Turn off the flame as soon as the milk heats. Stir while it's going to cool for a moment, and pour into a mug.

Step 3: Add honey, stir until well blended and enjoy your drink.

CHAPTER FOUR
BAKED GOODS

VATA BAKED GOODS

SODA BREAD

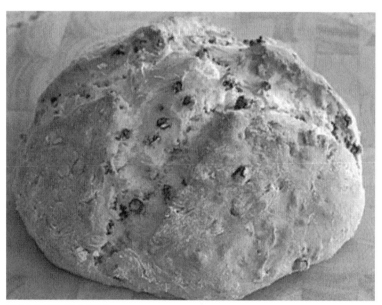

INGREDIENTS
- Walnuts 1/4cups, chopped water
- 1 cup, hot sugar
- 2 tablespoons Spelt flour
- ½ teaspoon Himalayan salt
- 5 teaspoons Oat flour

- 1/2 cups Baking soda
- 1 teaspoon Kefir milk,
- 1 cup Ghee
- 2 tablespoons Fennel seeds
- 4 Eggs
- dried carrots
- grilled baking powder 1 teaspoon

PREPARATIONS

Step 1: Soak diced eggs overnight in one cup of ho

Step 2: Put your spelt flour, oat flour, sucanate, baking powder, salt and fennel seeds in a medium-sized blending bowl. Mix them all very well.

Step 3: Heat ghee in a small bowl in a microwave oven.

Step 4: Put your kefir, almonds, grated carrots, ghee, dates and corresponding water in another medium bowl. Mix until it's all incorporated.

Step 5: Add the milk-fruit-nut-mixture to your dry bowl. Combine thoroughly with that. This is supposed to make a soda dough that is somewhat firm, but also slightly sticky. Apply a little more flour if you think it's required.

Step 6: Use a greased knife or your hands to break the dough into four or five pieces. Use your hands to make these pieces of dough into circular loaves approximately one inch high, and four or five inches in the middle.

Step 7: Gently position the shaped loaves on a baking sheet, the bottom of which is lined with parchment paper. Make sure to leave at least two inches of space between the loaves. It's possible to make a big loaf if you don't want to make separate batches of small ones.

Step 8: Bake in a pre-heated oven that is 375 degrees F for 30 to 40 minutes.

Step 9: Once removed from the oven, remove the baking sheet and place it on a refrigerator rack. When kept in a dry place, these breads can be packed in a clean towel. They're best served warm with ghee, though.

BERRY SCONES

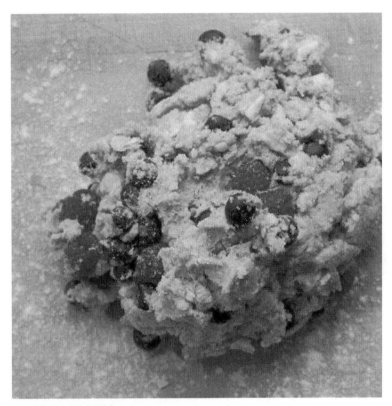

INGREDIENTS

- Blueberries
- 2 tablespoons fresh Mulberries
- 2 tablespoons fresh Coconut milk
- 1 cup chilled Ghee
- 3 tablespoons chilled Coconut blossom sugar
- 1 teaspoon Himalayan salt
- 5 teaspoons Baking Powder
- 1 tablespoon Oat Flour

- 1/3 cups Spelt flour

PREPARATIONS

Step 1: Get your food processor and add flours, salt, sugar and baking powder. Blend it until combined. Typically, this is done in just a few bursts.

Step2: Remove the cooled ghee and pump until the mixture has a sandy appearance with extremely fine crumbs.

Step 3: Quite gently, add the coconut milk, pour a little bit, then shake, then pour a little more. Do this until it starts to come together as a dough.

Step 4: Put the dough on a work surface that is thinly covered with oat or spelt flour. Gently fold the berries and knead them into the flour. Be careful you don't crush any of the fruit when you put it all together.

Step 5: Flatten dough up to an inch in height.

Step 6: Form into wedge forms. That's about eight scones.

Step 7: Put the wedges on a metal baking tray lined with parchment paper. If you want, brush a little coconut milk over the top of each and sprinkle with some coconut blossom sugar.

Step 8: Put the tray on the middle rack in an oven that has already been warmed to 375 degrees. Bake it until golden brown. It'll take around twenty to thirty minutes.

SESAME BREAD

INGREDIENTS

Sponge:

- Yeast, 1 teaspoon
- Dry Spelt Flour 2 cups
- Honey, 1 tablespoon
- fresh water, 1 cup, moist (not hot)

Dough:

- Sesame Seeds, 3 cups
- Himalayan Salt, pinch
- 2 cups Spelt Flour
- Honey, 1 tablespoon, raw

PREPARATIONS

Sponge:

Step 1: Dissolve raw honey in warm water. Stir in the yeast until it dissolves. To say if your water is too soft, put a clean finger in the bath. If it's not too dry, you'll be able to leave it there until the count of ten is reached, without it becoming too sticky. Set aside until the yeast begins to bubble and froth, which will take about 20 minutes.

Step 2: Add the two cups of spelt flour and beat with a whisk or an egg batter for one hundred strokes. This is the sponge of your bread.

Stage 3: Cover the bowl and allow the dough to stay in a warm place for about 40 minutes. It's expected to double in size next time.

DOUGH:

Step 1: Take your sponge and add the sesame, the Himalayan salt and two cups of the spelt flour. Mix well, guy.

Step 2: Flour should be added to your dough until it begins to draw away from the sides of the bowl, leaving the dough or extra flour to be clean or stray.

Step 3: Knead the dough for 10 minutes, still moving in the same direction. Sprinkle flour on the counter as needed to prevent the dough from sticking. Don't cheat on yourself and get out early; the full ten minutes are vital to making the dough reach its full potential.

Step 4: Put the dough in a warm, greased tub. Put a clean towel on top of your dish and put it in a warm place. Allow for forty minutes to interrupt. The mixture should be twice the original size by this point.

Step 5: When the dough is double its original size, pound the puffy center straight down.

Step 6: Cover the bowl and place it in a warm place for another forty minutes. Test the dough at the mark of forty minutes. It should be twice the size again. If not, quit for another twenty minutes.

Step 7: After the dough has risen in the bowl for a second time, pull it down again.

Step 8: Every enough dough in each muffin cup in a pre-fatted muffin pan to fill it half full.

Step 9: Let it climb to double the scale. It's only supposed to take about 20 minutes this period. You should preheat the oven to 350 degrees while it's going up.

Step 10: Put the oven preheated to 350 degrees F on the middle rack. Keep in the oven until golden brown, about 20 minutes.

PITTA BAKED GOODS

WALNUT BREAD

INGREDIENTS
- Yeast, 1 pack, dried Xantham Gum
- 1 teaspoon Walnuts
- 5 cups, minced Sorghum Flour
- ½ teaspoon Himalayan Salt
- 5 teaspoons Saffron

- 6 strands Turbinado Sugar
- 1/3 cups Potato Starch
- 1 cup Millet
- 1 cup Whole Organic Milk
- 5 cups Grass-fed Butter
- 5 cups, unsalted Water

PREPARATIONS

Step 1: Gently warm milk to just above room temperature. You can do this with a small saucepan over low heat or a microwave oven.

Step 2: In a small bowl, add warm milk, yeast and sugar. Cover the top of the bowl with a clean cloth and leave for 15 minutes.

Step3: Break the thread of a saffron with your hand or with a mortar and a pestle. Place in a small saucepan and cover with half a inch of boiling water. Set aside and let it go for five minutes.

Step 4: Put the chopped walnuts in a small bowl. Pour ample hot water to cover them. Set them aside and let them be there for now.

Step5: Using one of the larger mixing pots, combine rice, salt, starch, xantham gum and millet thoroughly.

Step6: Create a divot in the dry ingredients. Stir in the butter and the combination of the yeast. Make sure all the components are well mixed.

Step 7: Knead back and forth and side to side until the dough is running, smooth and no longer sticky. Once this point has been reached, roll it up into a ball and place it gently in a pre-greased bowl. Place a clean towel all over the place and let it be. Check in for two hours and make sure the place is heated enough. By this time, the dough was supposed to double in size. If not, leave for another thirty minutes, then check again.

Step 8: When your recipe has grown, the size of the recipe should be doubled. Punch it down and add some walnuts. Fold them in until they are evenly distributed throughout the flour.

Step9: Knead the dough for two to three minutes. Divide into two equal size lumps Step 10: flatten and roll up the jelly-roll style of the dough. Layer in pre-grained bread pans, cover the pans with clean towels. Let them be, and wait until your recipe reaches twice the size it was when you first put it in the pans. This is supposed to be about two hours.

Step 11: Cook until golden brown, in an oven that has been preheated to 400 degrees. It should take around twenty to twenty-five minutes.

CHAPATI

INGREDIENTS
- Sunflower oil, 2 teaspoons Water
- 1 teaspoon Himalayan salt
- ¼ teaspoons Flour
- 1 cup, whole-wheat pastry Spelt Flour

PREPARATIONS

Step 1: Place your flour, salt and water in a large mixing dish. Combine until the dough starts to form, then knead by hand or with a dough hook from the mixing machine.

Step 2: Mix in the sunflower oil and start to knead. Add more flour if you think it's necessary for the dough. This dough should not be hard, it should be workable, but it should be gentle.

Step 3: Using a greased knife or floured fingers, make twelve golf ball-sized dough balls out of the original large clump.

Step 4: Brush the surface of your job with dust. Take a dough ball and place it gently in the center of the floured field.

Step 5: Lightly powder your rolling pin, and continue to flatten your chapatti in the centre. This works best if you rotate a couple times, then switch, move, change 90 degrees, roll, and flip again. Keep until the chapatti is small enough, but it won't break as quickly as it is picked up. Make sure the dough is the same consistency all the way around and through.

Step 6: Put your flattened chapatti on a pre-heated griddle or skillet. Cast iron or a good quality non-stick pan is going to work the very best. The pan should be heated over medium-high, leaving the dough for thirty to sixty seconds.

Step 7: Flip the chapati after thirty to sixty seconds and flatten any bubbles that attempt to grow with the back of the spatula.

Step 8: Turn and click the chapatti twice until it is lightly browned on each hand.

Step 9: Clean and gently brush the molten ghee. Store in foil or in a large tortilla hot dish, however, they're best eaten fresh from the stovetop.

BANANA BREAD

INGREDIENTS
- Cardamom
- 5 teaspoons, ground cinnamon
- 1 teaspoon of coffee
- 1 teaspoon of walnuts
- 5 cups, minced baking powder
- 1 teaspoon of ripe bananas
- 3, mashed nutmeg
- 5 teaspoons, ground sugar
- 2, big honey
- 5 cups, fresh baking soda
- 1 teaspoon of sunflower oil
- 4 tablespoons of garlic
- 5 teaspoons, ground butter (unsalted)
- 4 tbsp, melted whole wheat.

PREPARATIONS

Step 1: Add the eggs while still beating the honey mixture. Make sure you add them one at a time, thoroughly integrating the first before opening the other.

Step 2: Remove cocoa and almonds, mix well.

Step 3: In a small medium-sized mixing bowl, whisk in the spelt, wheat and oat flour. Remove the spices and the leaven products, then mix properly.

Step 4: Mix the dry ingredients into a wet dough and apply all the components to the dough.

Step 5: Fold the mashed banana. Don't over-mix the beat.

Step 6: Spoon the batter into a pre-fatted bread pan or a pre-fatted muffin tray.

Step 7: Put a 350-degree pre-heated oven on the middle rack. Cook until a toothpick can be inserted in the center and pulled back with no dough stuck to it. It requires about 30 minutes.

Step 8: When the bread is completely baked, let it cool in the pan for five to ten minutes before removing it to the refrigerator. It's best served warm.

KAPHA BAKED GOODS

TEA CAKES–MADE WITH BUCKWHEAT, RASPBERRY AND ORANGE

- Yogurt 1/4 cups, plain vanilla
- 1 teaspoon, Turbinado Sugar extract
- 1/3 cups Strawberries
- 5 cups, fresh orange zest
- fresh eggs
- 3 Coconut Oil or Grass-fed butter
- 1/4 cups Buckwheat flour

PREPARATIONS

Step 1: Make sure your oven is set to 350 degrees Fahrenheit.

Step 2: Freely grease the 8x8 baking pan.

Step 3: Melt the butter or coconut oil in a small bowl or dish using a microwave.

Step 4: Beat eggs with an electric blender or with a vigorous arm and whisk. In small quantities, add the sugar to the eggs, whisking continuously. Keep whisking until the eggs are scrubbed.

Step 5: Beat the yogurt and vanilla extract in the egg mixture. Be sure to combine it completely.

Step 6: Remove the molten oil or butter quite gradually and start whisking until all is mixed.

Step 7: Apply flour in small quantities, slowly stirring until the mixture is smooth and pourable.

Step 8: Add the orange zest and fresh raspberries to the mixture.

Step 9: Leave the mixing bowl in the pre-fatted pan.

Step 10: Bake in the oven until the center is barely set, which is about thirty minutes away.

Step 11: Cool the oven for thirty minutes and cut into squares for a warm meal. Alternatively, instead, let it cool down absolutely and feed at room temperature.

ALMOND-QUINOA BREAD

INGREDIENTS

- apple cider vinegar
- tablespoon Coconut oil
- 5 fresh Egg
- 1/5 teaspoon Himalayan salt
- 1/4 teaspoons Maple syrup
- 1 tablespoon Soda
- 5 teaspoons Coconut flour
- 2 teaspoons Arrowroot powder
- 2 tablespoons Flaxseed meal
- ¼ cups Quinoa flour
- 5 cups Almond flour

PREPARATIONS

Step 1: Remove 5 eggs, coconut oil, maple syrup and vinegar. Blend until fully blended with the pulse settings.

Step 2: When the batter is completely mixed, increasing it in a pan lined with parchment paper.

Step 3: Position on the middle rack of an oven that has been preheated to 350 degrees. Aim for a golden brown top and a clean toothpick from the middle to see if it's finished. It takes between twenty-five to thirty-five minutes.

Step 4: When the loaf is sufficiently baked, remove it from the oven, but do not remove the bread from the pan. Let the loaf chill for at least one hour before you try to put it on a cooling rack to finish the cooling. Before cutting, the bread should be completely cool.

TEFF BREAD

INGREDIENTS
- Butter
- 1 tablespoon Baking powder
- 1.5 teaspoons Coconut oil
- 1/2 tablespoon Himalayan salt
- 1/4 teaspoons Bacon,
- 1 basil
- 1 teaspoon, infinite choices–experiment Apple Cider Vinegar
- 1 teaspoon (optional) Teff flour

PREPARATIONS

Step 1: Put vinegar, oil, bacon, salt, flour and baking powder in a medium-sized mixing bowl, and com.

Step 2: Allow the batter to rest for 2 minutes.

Step 3: Put the tablespoon of butter in a skillet that has been preheated over a medium - high burner. Let it melt away.

Step 4: Scrape the dough into the frying pan and leave until it appears to have risen slightly. It'll take about two to three minutes. Flip the bread over when it reaches this point.

Step 5: Cook bread on this side for two to three minutes, too.

Step 6: Remove the bread pan from the heat. Slice into the wedges and serve with a stuffed dip.

CHAPTER FIVE
SOUPS

VATA SOUPS

POTATO FENNEL SOUP

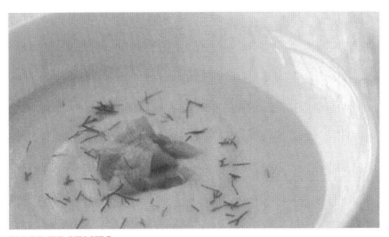

INGREDIENTS
- 2 cups Water
- 6 cups Sunflower oil
- 1/2 tablespoons Himalayan salt
- 5 teaspoons Red pepper
- ¼ teaspoons Potatoes
- 4 Peeled and chopped Leeks
- 1 cup, chopped Fennel seeds
- 1 tablespoon Black Pepper

PREPARATION

Step 1: In a medium-sized pot, pour four cups of water. Add the chopped potatoes and boil for 10 minutes.

Step 2: After the potatoes are boiled, take the potatoes out of the boiling water and place them in two cups of cool water. Keep the hot water in your pot.

Step 3: Strain the potatoes out of the cool water and place them in the blender. Blend until it's perfect.

Step 4: Return the now-purified potatoes to a pot of hot water and bring them back to a boil.

Step 5: Add the leeks, fennel, peppers, salt and oil when the water boils. Stir well, turn the heat to weak.

Step 6: Simmer for at least 20 minutes and serve hot.

LIGHT CABBAGE SOUP

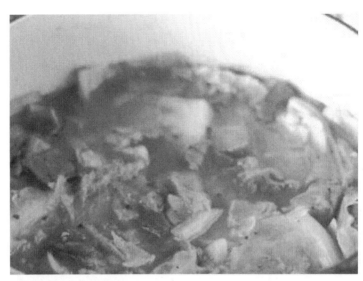

INGREDIENTS

- Yellow Onion
- 1/4 teaspoon Himalayan Salt
- 5 teaspoons Parsley
- 1/4 cups, fresh Garlic
- 1 clove, minced Curry Powder
- 1/4 teaspoons Celery
- 1/4 cups Cabbage,
- 4 cups, cooked Black Pepper, to taste

PREPARATIONS

Step 1: Place all ingredients together in a large pot.

Step 2: Pour in enough water to cover all of the ingredients. Give a quick swirl.

Step 3: Put the pot on a high heat until it boils. Reduce heat to low after boiling. Cover and start to cook the broth.

Step4: Simmer broth for at least 45 minutes. The vegetables are expected to be tender.

CHICKEN RICE SOUP

INGREDIENTS

- Pinch Yellow Onion
- 5 cups, chopped water
- 1/6 teaspoon Himalayan salt
- 5 teaspoons Chicken meat
- 1/4 pounds, chopped celery
- 5 cups, chopped carrots
- 4, chopped black pepper
- 1 teaspoon of basmati rice
- 1 cup Ginger, pinch Cumin

PREPARATIONS

Step 1: Place each ingredient in another large pot.

Step 2: Take the mixture to a simmer, use a burner set to extreme, and swirl again and again.

Step 3: When the kettle is heating, turn the heat down until the liquid is simmering. Simmer for an hour.
Step 4: Eat yourself nice and enjoy!

CARROT SOUP

INGREDIENTS
- ¼ teaspoon Himalayan salt
- 1/4 teaspoons Olive oil
- 2 teaspoons Ginger
- 1 teaspoon, freshly ground celery
- 2 tablespoons, roughly chopped carrots
- 2, roughly chopped black pepper

PREPARATIONS
Step 1: Place chopped carrots, chopped celery and ginger in a high powered blender. Puree until the silk is clean.
Step 2: Measure the filtered mixture into a medium bath. Remove the pepper and the salt and the butter. Bring to a boil for 10 to 15 minutes.

PITTA SOUPS

MINT BEET SOUP

INGREDIENTS
- 1 cup, finely chopped Sugar
- 1/5 teaspoon Himalayan salt
- ¼ teaspoons Mint
- 1/4 cups, fresh, pure Ginger
- 1 tsp, freshly ground Ghee
- 2 tablespoons Black pepper
- ¼ teaspoons Beets

PREPARATIONS

Step 1: Puree beets, water, pepper, salt and ginger, using a food processor or blender.

Step 2: Pour into a medium sauce pan. Add it and stir in the ghee.

Step 3: Frequently stirring, boiling. Continue cooking at a simmer, turn the heat to low. Cook until thick, stirring now and then to avoid burning.

Step 4: Add the purified mint leaves to the soup 10 minutes before the burner is removed.

MUSHROOM AND ASPARAGUS CREAM

PREPARATIONS

- 1 cupYellow onion
- 1/4 cups, chopped thyme
- 2 teaspoons, fresh Himalayan sal
- ¼ teaspoons Garlic
- 1 clove, minced mushrooms
- 1/5 cups, crimini and a circle, finely sliced sugar
- 2 tablespoons, unsalted black pepper
- 1/4 teaspoons Asparagus
- 2 cups Blanched almonds

PREPARATIONS

Step 1: heat one tablespoon of unsalted butter, sauté. Once done, remove from the pan and set aside for the time being.

Step 2: Place the finely sliced mushrooms in the bottom of the pan with the remaining tablespoon of oil. Be sure they're not going to strike. Mushrooms are too close together to steam each other with a evaporating water vapor instead of sautéing.

Step 3: Put salt, asparagus, pepper, onion, garlic, thyme and white almonds in a blender or food processor. Add a cup of water and a little purée. Attach small amounts of water if needed to ensure a smooth blending operation. Keep in mind that nuts blend better in a thicker base liquid, and you can add more water once they're all in the pot.

Step 4: Once the soup has been properly blended, pour it into a medium-sized pot. Pour enough water to make the consistency you want. Simmer for a couple of minutes.

COLD CUCUMBER LIME SOUP

INGREDIENTS
- 1 tablespoon of Himalayan salt
- 1/4 teaspoons Lime
- 1/5 juice Lemon
- 1 teaspoon, freshly ground Cucumber
- 2 cups, finely diced Cilantro,
- 2 cups sunflower oil

PREPARATIONS

Step 1: mix cilantro and lemon in a blender or in a food processor. Strain out all the chunks.

Step 2: Apply the finely diced cucumber to the coriander and mix well.

Step3: Blend the lime juice, salt and oil properly.

Step 4: Serve with coconut shavings, bean sprouts or mint leaves.

KAPHA SOUPS

TURMERIC VEGETABLE SOUP

INGREDIENTS
- Water, enough to cover the ingredients
- filtered Zucchini
- 1, chopped Yellow Onio
- 5 cups, chopped Sunflower oil
- 2 tablespoons of Sucanate
- 1 tablespoon of Black Pepper

- 5 teaspoons of Turmeric
- 1 teaspoon of Potatoes
- 2, peeled and diced Mustard seed
- 1/5 teaspoons of ground Mung beans
- 1/5 teaspoon Himalayan salt
- 1 teaspoon of Lime,

PREPARATIONS

Step 1: Remove the other spices then remove some water to the spices. This water is drained by the ground spices and forms a paste. Allow the paste to remain alone for at least five minutes.

Step 2: Place one tablespoon of sunflower oil in a small pan. When it's hot, add the spices that are now in paste form. Sauté for the next thirty seconds. Make sure you don't let the spices brown or lose their taste. Turn the burner off and set it aside.

Step 3: In a large pot, boil another tablespoon of sunflower oil. Attach the sliced yellow onion and sauté until it is transparent.

Step 4: Remove the garlic once the onion has become translucent. Fry the garlic for thirty seconds, stirring to prevent burning.

Step 5: Now transfer the spices from the small pan to the large pot and mix well.

Step 6: Add the zucchini, carrots, lime juice, beans, ginger, potatoes and sugar. Cover with some water.

Step 7: Place the pot full of goodness on high heat until it boils. Once the soup is boiling, cover with a lid and turns the heat to low. Let the soup boil in the ingredients, which will take about an hour.

Step 8: Serve in a small bowl of cilantro, lime and coconut.

BARLEY MERLOT SOUP

INGREDIENTS
- 1/4 teaspoon Himalayan salt
- 5 teaspoons Rosemary
- 2 teaspoons Merlot
- 1 cup Coriander seeds
- 1 teaspoon Ghee
- 2 tablespoons Garlic
- 1 Clove, minced Mushrooms
- 1 cup Crimini and Button
- sliced Black Pepper
- 1/4 teaspoons Barley

- 1/5 cups, coarsely ground or whole yellow onions

PREPARATIONS

Step 1: When pan is hot, sauté the barley in the ghee until it starts to smell nutty or roasted.

Step 2: Boil up to 6 cups of water. Remove the barley and the ghee.

Step 3: Add salt to boiling water and stir again and again, heating until the barley is tender.

Step 4: Take your ground coriander and sauté it in the next tablespoon of ghee.

Step 5: Remove the chopped crimini and button mushrooms and the chopped onion to the ghee. Sauté until it browns.

Step 6: When the onions and mushrooms are browned, introduce the garlic and rosemary.

Step 7: Apply the coriander-mushroom-onion-mixture to the water once the barley is properly softened. Stir it together.

Step 8: When all is well balanced, shut off the burner and remove the pot from the flame.

Step 9: Remove the wine and mix well immediately before eating this soup.

FENNEL CORN SOUP

INGREDIENTS
- 1 tablespoon of Himalayan salt
- 1/4 teaspoons Fennel seeds
- 5 teaspoons, ground with mortar and pestle Rice
- 4 cups, purified Corn meal
- 1 cup, sunflower oil

PREPARATION

Step 1: Blend cornmeal and rice with a medium-sized bowl. Use a burner set to extreme, bring to a boil. When the corn meal is hot, turn the heat to low and start to simmer

Step 2: add salt, ground fennel and oil to the soup and mix until well blended.

Step 3: Simmer for another 20 minutes. Serve hot with a garnish of corn and parsley.

CHAPTER SIX
STEWS AND KITCHARIS

VATA STEWS AND KITCHARIS

POMEGRANATE STEW

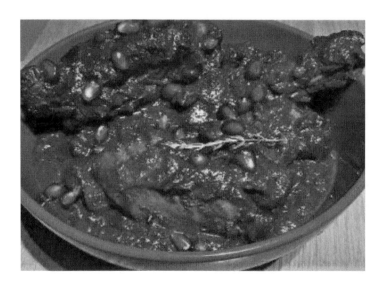

INGREDIENTS
- 1Cup Walnuts
- 1.5 cups, Toasted Turmeric
- 1/5 teaspoons Himalayan salt,
- ¼ teaspoons Pomegranate juice

- 1 cup Maple syrup
- 1 tablespoon Ghee
- 2 tablespoons Cinnamon
- 1/4 teaspoons, ground Chicken
- 2 pounds, breasts and thighs Black Pepper
- 1/4teaspoons Chicken Broth
- 1-3 cups yellow onions

PREPARATIONS

Step 1: Place pomegranate juice in a small sauce. Set a low simmering burner for thirty minutes. Set it to the side.

Step2: Take your toasted walnuts and break them into very fine pieces using a food processor.

Step 3: Heat one tablespoon of the ghee over a medium-high burner using your dutch oven. In the ghee, sauté meat, sprinkle with salt gently. Take it out of the pan when the chicken is cooked through.

Step 4: Put the onions and another tablespoon of ghee in a hot dutch oven. Reduce to medium heat.

Step 5: When the onions are clear, place the chicken back in the pot. Add enough broth to give the desired consistency.

Step 6: Heat to boil. Turn the heat to weak and simmer. Mix thoroughly in raw walnuts, sugar, pomegranate, cinnamon, pepper, turmeric and oil.

Step 7: Simmer for thirty to forty minutes.

KOMBU KITCHARI

INGREDIENTS

Kombu,

- 1 stick Turmeric
- 5 teaspoons, Hing
- 1/4 teaspoons Himalayan salt
- 5 teaspoons Ginger
- 1 teaspoon, freshly ground cumin seeds
- 1 teaspoon Ghee
- 3 tablespoons Oil
- 4 cups Black mustard seeds
- 1 teaspoon Mung beans
- 5 cups Basmati rice

PREPARATIONS

Step 1: Rinse rice and beans and soak overnight. Oh, dump.

Step 2: Steam the ghee in a medium saucepan. Sauté the garlic, the cumin, the ginger and the pepper for a few minutes

Step 3: Add your four cups of water to this mixture and turn the heat up to high. Just stir occasionally.

Step 4: Once your kitchari is boiling, apply the kombu handle, salt, turmeric and ing. Stir well and lower the fire.

Step 5: Cover, cook for thirty to forty minutes, or until all the ingredients in your meal are soft. Pay attention, as more small amounts of water may need to be added to prevent burning.

Step 6: Serve hot, garnished with coriander.

CHILI–LENTIL AND RICE

INGREDIENTS

- Himalayan salt, pinch
- 1/4 teaspoons Black pepper
- Pinch Mustard,
- 1/8 teaspoons, dried Paprika
- 1/2 teaspoons Cumin
- 1/2 teaspoons Chili powder
- 1/5 teaspoons Butter
- 5 teaspoons Sweet Red Pepper
- 25 diced Carrot
- 1, diced Celery
- 1 seed, diced Ghee
- 1 tablespoon Bragg Liquid Aminos

- 1 tablespoon Bay Leaf
- 1, dry Vegetable or Bone Broth

PREPARATIONS

Step 1: Heat the ghee in a medium sized bowl. In the heated ghee, sauté all the vegetables until soft

Step 2: When the vegetables are tender, add the rice, lentils, braggs and bay leaf. Just sauté for another minute or two

Step 3: Add the broth to the pot and stir to ensure that everything is well integrated. Bring it to a boil.

Step 4: After boiling, reduce the heat and simmer the chili until the rice and lentils are soft and tender.

Phase 5: Serve with some sour cream and cheese.

PITTA STEWS AND KITCHARIS

COCONUT AND CILANTRO KITCHARI

INGREDIENTS
- 6 cups Turmeric
- 1/5 teaspoons Himalayan salt
- 1/4 teaspoons Mung beans

- 5 cups, cut and dried Ginger
- 2 teaspoons Ghee
- 2 tablespoons Coconut flakes
- 1/3 cups Cilantro
- 3 cups, fresh Basmati rice
- 1 cup sugar

PREPARATIONS

Step 1: Rinse beans and rice. Put the mung beans and the rice in the bath for a few hours.

Step 2: Clean the beans and the pasta.

Step 3: In a blender, puree ginger, almond, half a cup of water and cilantro.

Step 4: Heat the ghee in a medium-sized pot and whisk in the distilled mixture of coconut, turmeric and salt. Bring to a boil, stirring frequently.

Step 5: Remove 6 cups of water. It's Heat. Add the rice and the mung beans, then mix them.

Step 6: Take all of this to a boil again and simmer for five minutes. Lower the heat of the flame and protect your kitchari.

Step 7: Simmer for 20 to 30 minutes or until all is tender.

Vegetable Stew

INGREDIENTS

- Black pepper
- tiny pinch of Himalayan salt
- 1 teaspoon of water
- 7 cups Carrots
- 3, diced Broccoli
- 1 small head, chopped celery
- 5 stalks, diced New potatoes
- 6 thin, quartered Corn
- 2 legs, fresh Coriander seed
- 5 teaspoons, freshly ground Fennel seed,
- ¼ teaspoons, freshly ground Extra virgin olive oil
- 1 tablespoon Cumin
- 1/4 teaspoons, ground anise

PREPARATIONS

Step 1: Using high heat to bring in the anise. As soon as the anise begins to pop, extract the heat and stir in the remaining spices.

Step 2: Cut the corn out of the cob.

Step 3: Add all the vegetables in the pot. Place again over high heat and add seven cups of water.

Step 4: Bring the pot to a rolling boil, reduce the heat to medium / medium-high and cover.

Step 5: Boil the stew for twenty to twenty-five minutes until all the vegetables are tender.

TURMERIC MUNG BEAN STEW

INGREDIENTS

- 1 head, diced Lemons
- 2, juiced Black pepper
- 1/5 teaspoons Himalayan salt
- 1 teaspoon Ginger
- 1 tablespoon, freshly ground Turmeric
- 1/5 teaspoons Cumin
- 1 teaspoon, ground water
- 6 cups Coriander
- 1 teaspoon, ground Mung beans
- 1 cup Celery
- 4 stalks, diced Carrots
- 4, peeled and diced Ghee
- 1 tablespoon kale

PREPARATIONS

Step 1: Soak mung beans

Step 2: Place ghee in a large stock pot and heat with medium heat.

Step 3: Sauté the spices until the fragrant aromas are released.

Step 4: Remove the beans, carrots and celery to the hot ghee and sauté the celery is tender.

Step 5: Add 6 cups of water and lemon juice. Take it to a simmer.

Step 6: When the stew cooks, reduce the heat to simmer and cover.

Step 7: Cook until vegetables and beans are tender and soft. It takes about twenty to thirty minutes.

Step 8: Add your kale. Simmer until wilted, about one to two minutes.

Step 9: Serve hot, topped with fresh parsley and cilantro.

KAPHA STEWS AND KITCHARIS

MUNG BEAN KITCHARI

INGREDIENTS
- Water, 4 cups, plus more for soaking and boiling beans
- Pinch Himalayan salt
- ¼ teaspoons Mung beans

- 5 cups, split beans Ginger
- 1 tablespoon, freshly ground Ghee
- 2 tablespoons Cumin
- 1 teaspoon, ground Cloves
- 1/4 teaspoons, ground Cinnamon
- ¼ teaspoons, ground Cardamom
- 1/4 teaspoons, ground Bay leaves
- 4, dry Basmati rice

PREPARATIONS

Step 1: Soak the rice for a few hours and drain.

Step 2: Place the mung beans and the rice in a pot with six cups of water. Remove the leaves of the harbor. Put the pot on the burner and turn the heat up high. When the beans and water begin to simmer, scrape some foam off the surface with a spoon and dump it. Boil for 3 to 5 minutes.

Step 3: Lift the beans and the rice out of the water and put them back in the pot. Add four cups of fresh water.

Step 4: Simmer the beans for one to three hours or until they disintegrate in the bath with the pasta.

Step 5: Mix all the spices with a small amount of water and let it rest for five minutes.

Step 6: Heat the ghee in a large non-stick pan and sauté the spices until they begin to be aromatic.

Step 7: Pour a quarter of a cup of water into the pan, stir to make sure all the flavours, and add the mung beans and the rice.

Step 8: Simmer for 20 to 30 minutes and serve hot.

RED CABBAGE STEW

INGREDIENTS
- 1/4 teaspoon Himalayan salt
- 1/5 teaspoons of olive oil
- 2 tablespoons of brown sugar
- 2 tablespoons of red cabbage
- 4 cups of apple cider vinegar
- 1/4 cups of black pepper
- 5 teaspoons yellow onions

PREPARATIONS

Step 1: Slice both pieces into thin slices, resulting in a small amount of cabbage.

Step 2: Place the chopped cabbage in a large pot with enough water to cover it. Steam to simmer. Lowering the sun, keep simmering.

Step 3: In a small saucepan, sauté the onion in the olive oil until the onion is soft and transparent. Apply the vinegar and whisk when the onion becomes transparent.

Step 4: Add the onion and vinegar to the boiling pot of the cabbage. Stir until the water is well mixed.

Step 5: Apply brown sugar, salt and pepper to the mixture. Keep simmering, protected with the bowl, until all is tender. Serve yourself hot.

VEGGIE STEW

INGREDIENTS
- Himalayan salt, pinch
- 5 teaspoons Cayenne pepper
- Pinch Black pepper
- pinch Ginger
- 2 teaspoons, freshly ground Fennel seeds
- 1 teaspoon, ground Coriander seeds
- 5 teaspoons, ground Cumin
- 5 teaspoons, ground Turmeric

- 5 teaspoons, ground Basil
- 5 teaspoons, dried Apple Cider vinegar
- 2 tablespoons Sesame oil
- 2 tablespoons Tomato,

PREPARATIONS

Step 1: Add the water. Vegetables and liquid should be held a few centimeters below the rim of the bottle.

Step 2: Mix in all of the spices.

Step 3: Remove the oil and mix it.

Step 4: Place the lid on the crockpot and turn the heat to a low setting. You know, make sure it's low and not just dry.

Step 5: Leave for 8 to 10 hours.

Step 6: When the stew is done, add the vinegar, the pepper and the salt as desired. Serve yourself heavy.

CHAPTER SEVEN
VEGETABLES, GRAINS, AND LEGUMES

VATA VEGETABLES, GRAINS, AND LEGUMES

COCONUT RICE

INGREDIENTS
- 1/3 teaspoon Himalayan salt
- 1/4 teaspoons Coconut oil
- 2 tablespoons Coconut flakes
- 5 cups Basmati Rice, 1 cup water

PREPARATIONS

Step 1: Boil water in a medium saucepan.

Step 2: Toast half of the coconut flakes and set aside.

Step 3: Mix in the boiling water the sugar, half of the coconut flakes (1/4 cups), salt and oil. Bring water to a boil again.

Step 4: When the water is boiling again, lower the heat and cover. Simmer till the rice is tender.

Step 5: Serve hot and garnished with toasted coconut flakes.

Roasted Sweet Potato with Kale

INGREDIENTS
- Sweet Potato
- 2 cups Ghee
- 1 teaspoon Himalayan salt
- ¼ teaspoons Kale
- 5 pounds minced Ginger, 1.5 teaspoons
- freshly ground water, for boiling

PREPARATIONS

Step 1: Put Kale in boiling water and cook until it has rendered a lovely and bright green hue.

Step 2: In an additional pot, dump the sweet potatoes and salt. Water should be added until all of it is covered. Heat to boil and continue to boil until the sweet potatoes are soft with a fork

Step 3: When the potatoes are done, drain them out of the water and set aside.

Step 4: Heat ghee in a medium-sized pan with a medium - high flame. Wait until the ghee is hot, and then add the ginger. Sauté for the next thirty seconds

Step 5: Add the potatoes and the kale to the hot ginger ghee and mix carefully, as you don't want to break the tender potatoes apart.

Step 6: Serve yourself hot.

SQUASH TAHINI SALAD

- Tahini,
- 1/3 teaspoons Himalayan salt
- 5 teaspoons Red onion
- 3 tablespoons, raw and diced Parsley
- ¼ cups, fresh, chopped Olive oil
- 1/4 cups Lime,
- 1, juice Garlic
- 2 cloves, minced Chickpeas
- 1 cup of canned Butternut squash
- 3 cups, sliced, de-pulped, and chopped

PREPARATIONS

Step 1: rinse chickpeas, save two tablespoons of bean juice

Step 2: Carefully combine one clove of garlic with two tablespoons of olive oil and half of the salt (.25 teaspoons). Remove the squash, whisk again.

Step 3: On a baking sheet with edges, cover the bottom with parchment paper. Attach the cooked squash to the pan and toast in a hot oven for at least 15 minutes, swirling the squash and rotating the pan halfway through. Remove when the squash is soft and tender.

Step 4: As the squash is frying, you should put the tahini, the remaining garlic clove, the lemon juice, the olive oil (two tablespoons), the bean juice that you saved, and the remaining 25 teaspoons of salt in the blender. Puree deeply and dump it into a bowl.

Step 5: Rinse and rinse the diced onion.

Step 6: Blend the onion and the parsley and the tahini.

Step 7: Mix the roasted squash into the prepared tahini and serve immediately.

PITTA VEGETABLES, GRAINS AND LEGUMES

STIR FRY WITH RICE

- 1 tablespoon, finely chopped Turmeric
- ¼ teaspoons, ground Cumin
- 1/4 teaspoons, ground Coriander seeds
- 1/4 teaspoons, ground Fennel seeds
- ¼ teaspoons, ground Cardamom
- 1/4 teaspoons, ground Carrot
- 1, peeled and grated Zucchini
- 1, peeled and grated Cabbage
- 1.5 cups, minced rice
- 2 cups mint leaves

PREPARATIONS

Step 1: Heat one tablespoon of oil in a frying pan or a small wok. When heated, add a pinch of salt to the rice and sauté until it is clear.

Step 2: Spoon the water over the now transparent rice and boil until the rice has absorbed all the water. It's going to be about fifteen minutes.

Step 3: Heat the remaining four tablespoons of oil in a separate pan. When it's hot, stir in all the seasonings and sauté until the delicious aroma is released.

Step 4: In a spicy pan, dump the grated carrot and the zucchini and the chopped cabbage. Stir constantly and simmer for 10 minutes.

Step 5: Combine the vegetables with the rice. Season to taste, drink hot and enjoy it.

CARROT SALAD

INGREDIENTS

- 4 Raisin
- 1/4 cups Orange blossom water
- 5 teaspoons Grapefruit
- 5 cups, cut into chunks Carrots

PREPARATIONS

Step 1: Mix all ingredients in a medium sized mixing bowl. If the mixture is too dry, add a small amount of the juice you want.

Quinoa Cucumber Salad

INGREDIENTS

- 1 teaspoon Himalayan salt
- Quinoa dash
- 5 cups, pre-cooked Lime zest
- 5 teaspoons Lime
- 5, cups Kale juice
- ¼ pounds, chopped Cucumber
- 5 cups, water

PREPARATIONS

Step 1: Make sure your quinoa is chilled or room-temperature.

Step 2: Steam your chopped kale for about ten minutes and then take it out of the heat.

Step 3: Mix the diced cucumber and the steamed kale. Remove the zest of lime and just remove it.

Stage 4: Combine all components slowly and carefully. Serve chilled or at room temperature.

KAPHA VEGETABLES, GRAINS, AND LEGUMES

CINNAMON LENTILS AND RICE

INGREDIENTS

- yellow onion
- 1/4 cups, diced Walnuts,
- garnished Parsley,
- garnished Garlic 2 cloves
- pinch Himalayan salt
- 5 teaspoons Olive oil
- 3 tablespoons Lemon
- ¼ teaspoon juiced Cumin
- 1 teaspoon, ground Brown lentils
- 1/4 cups Black Pepper
- 5 cups Basmati rice, 1 cup Cinnamon
- 2 cups water

PREPARATIONS

Step 1: Use your wok to heat olive oil in preparation for sautéing. Add the onion to the oil and sauté for three or four minutes.

Step 2: Add garlic and sauté for 30 seconds.

Step 3: Add rice and sauté until it starts to turn brown.

Step 54Strain the lentils and incorporate the cabbage, rice and garlic. Combine thoroughly with that.

Step 6: Incorporate the lemon juice, salt, cumin, cinnamon and black pepper. Add the water and heat to the boil.

Step 7: When it boils, turn the mixture down and simmer until the rice is done. Serve hot with walnuts and parsley.

CILANTRO AND CORIANDER CORN

INGREDIENTS
- 1/5 teaspoon Himalayan salt
- ¼ teaspoons Lemon
- 5, Corn cobs,
- 4, chopped and de-silked Coriander seeds
- 1 tablespoon, ground with coffee grinder or mortar Cilantro
- 1/4 cups, fresh, chopped Ghee

PREPARATIONS

Step 1: Put the corn in boiling water and leave for 10 minutes.

Step2: Blend the cilantro, coriander and salt in the ghee.

Step 3: Pack the corn while it's still hot and serve immediately.

TOMATO FAVA BEAN SALAD

INGREDIENTS
- Tomatoes, 2, chopped Tahini
- 1 teaspoon of Himalayan salt
- 5 teaspoons Red onion
- 5 cups, diced Parsley
- 1/4 cups, fresh, chopped Olive oil
- 2 tablespoons of Lemon
- 1 tablespoon of Fava beans
- 1 cup, dried Cumin
- 2 teaspoons, ground Chickpeas
- 1 cup of Water, 4 cups

PREPARATIONS

Step 1: Place the chopped tomatoes in a saucepan and heat to boil. Boil, stirring frequently, until it is reduced to a thick sauce

Step 2: Heat one tablespoon of olive oil with your frying pan on a medium - high flame. Stir in the onion and sauté until the mixture is transparent. This takes only five minutes.

Step 3: Add the garlic and sauté for another thirty seconds.

Step 4: Apply fava beans and salt to the garlic and onion. Stir well and sauté for a couple of seconds. Pour four cups of water over everything, mix well, and turn the burner down to simmer for three hours. Beans are not expected to have a chalky middle.

Step 5: Once the beans are finished, strain them out of the liquid and boil until only 1 cup of water remains.

Step 6: Put the fava bean back in the pot. Attach the tomato sauce, tahini, lemon juice, and cumin to match. Simmer for about five minutes.

Step 7: Puree the entire dish with a blender or a food processor. Serve hot or chilled with parsley, onion or oil as a garnish.

CONCLUSION

The Ayurvedic diet is a meal plan based on the principles of Ayurvedic medicine, a type of traditional medicine that dates back millennia.

The diet involves eating or restricting certain foods on the basis of your dosha or type of body, which is claimed to increase weight loss and support attention.

It can be confusing and restrictive though, and it's based on subjective assumptions about your personality and type of body. Plus, scientific evidence does not back up its theories.

Ayurvedic lifestyle is one that improves your health, gives you well-being and helps to relieve your stress. The recipes in this book have been chosen with the utmost care to help you find balanced energy, and I hope that they will bring harmony and joy to your table and your life. I hope you've found a number of recipes in this cookbook to please your palate. Thank you for including me on your ayurvedic journey.

Printed in Great Britain
by Amazon

42760702R00079